The American
Diabetes Association®

The American
Dietetic Association

FAMILY
COOKBOOK

Volume IV

Also by the authors from SIMON & SCHUSTER

The American Diabetes Association
The American Dietetic Association
Family Cookbook, Volume I (Revised Edition)

The American Diabetes Association
The American Dietetic Association
Family Cookbook, Volume II (Revised Edition)

The American Diabetes Association
The American Dietetic Association
Family Cookbook, Volume III

The American Diabetes Association
Holiday Cookbook
Betty Wedman, M.S., R.D.

The American Diabetes Association
Special Celebrations and Parties Cookbook
Betty Wedman, M.S., R.D.

The American Diabetes Association®

The American Dietetic Association

FAMILY COOKBOOK

Volume IV

With Microwave Adaptations

Illustrated by Lauren Jarrett

SIMON AND SCHUSTER
New York · London · Toronto · Sydney · Tokyo · Singapore

SIMON & SCHUSTER
Simon & Schuster Building
Rockefeller Center
1230 Avenue of the Americas
New York, New York 10020

Library of Congress Cataloging-in-Publication Data is available.

ISBN: 0-671-76695-3

Designed by Rhea Braunstein

Manufactured in the United States of America

5   7   9   10   8   6   4

Acknowledgments

The American Diabetes Association and The American Dietetic Association gratefully acknowledge the following contributors:

Recipe Development:
Karen Levin
Recipe Testing:
Pat Dailey
Nutrition Analysis and Exchange Calculations:
Madelyn L. Wheeler, M.S., R.D., C.D.E.
Lawrence A. Wheeler, M.D., Ph.D.

Technical Reviewers:
Mary Carey, Ph.D., R.D.
Anne Daly, M.S., R.D., C.D.E.
Harold Holler, R.D., C.D.E.
Margaret D. Simko, Ph.D., R.D.
Madelyn L. Wheeler, M.S., R.D., C.D.E.

Text Writer/Editor:
Dorothy H. Segal

Manuscript Production:
Susan Hayes Coughlin
Deborah L. McBride
Barbara J. Sutcliffe

Contents

Foreword

America's historical role as the "melting pot" for people of many nationalities has contributed to the development of a rich and varied cuisine. Americans from the earliest settlers to the latter-day immigrants all brought cultural and culinary traditions that were transformed by the native peoples and foodstuffs of the new land. As America grew and the new arrivals took root, various cooking styles blossomed in different regions of the country. Today, this rich heritage is uniquely American.

Recently, the term "regional cooking" has taken on new meaning as a new generation of creative young chefs carries on the tradition of creating uniquely American cuisine, with cooking methods and ingredients blended from many different nationalities and cultures. This cookbook takes its cue from both the traditional dishes of the country's regions and the new American cuisine.

Today, too, the emphasis is shifting to the freshest, purest—and healthiest—ingredients and cooking techniques, a reflection of the new American life-style that focuses on nutrition and fitness as the keystones of good health. This cookbook capitalizes on today's emphasis on health and fitness by providing delicious, nutritious recipes for the entire family.

The American Diabetes Association and The American Dietetic Association are proud to join in presenting Volume IV of our Family Cookbook series. Like its predecessors, the recipes in this book follow nutrition guidelines developed by our two organizations for people with diabetes. However, it is important to note that these guidelines closely parallel the type of diet now recommended by the federal government and various health agencies for all of us. People with diabetes have been following these recommendations for years, and it is gratifying to see the rest of America beginning to follow suit!

This cookbook gives you a taste of the best of American regional cooking—with recipes specially developed to meet today's goals for healthy eating.

JAY S. SKYLER, M.D.
President
The American Diabetes Association

MARY ABBOTT HESS, M.S., R.D.
President
The American Dietetic Association

About the Associations

The American Diabetes Association (ADA) is the nation's leading voluntary health organization dedicated to improving the well-being of all people affected by diabetes. Equally important is its unceasing support for research to prevent and cure this chronic disease that affects some 14 million Americans. The Association carries out this important mission through the efforts of thousands of volunteers working at state affiliates and local chapters in more than 800 communities throughout the United States.

Membership in the American Diabetes Association puts you in contact with a network of more than 270,000 caring people throughout the country. Affiliates and chapters offer support groups, educational programs, counseling, and other special services. Membership also brings twelve issues of the lively patient education magazine, *Diabetes Forecast.*

In addition, the Association publishes an array of materials for every age group on topics important not just to the individual with diabetes, but to the entire family. Considerable effort is also devoted to educating health-care professionals and building public awareness about diabetes.

The American Diabetes Association also distributes a free, quarterly newsletter with practical advice and helpful hints on living with diabetes. To receive a copy, just call the toll-free number listed below.

Information on ADA membership and programs is available through the state affiliates (listed in the white pages of the telephone book) or through The American Diabetes Association, Inc.®, Diabetes Information Service Center, 1660 Duke Street, Alexandria, VA 22314; 1-800-ADA-DISC.

The American Dietetic Association is the nation's largest group of food and nutrition professionals with nearly 60,000 members. Its goal is to promote optimal health and nutritional status for Americans. The National Center for Nutrition and Dietetics is the public education initiative of The American Dietetic Association and its Foundation. The Center sponsors a series of programs to inform and educate the public about food and nutrition issues. The Center is housed in The American Dietetic Association building at 216 W. Jackson Blvd., Chicago, IL 60606-6995.

The ADA is dynamic as are its members—changing, adapting, and responding to new scientific findings and practical nutritional needs of the nation's people. The ADA members—with extensive scientific background—apply knowledge of food, nutrition, biochemistry, physiology, management, and behavioral and social sciences to promote health, prevent disease, and speed recovery from illness.

Most members are registered dietitians (R.D.) who have completed at least a bachelor's degree and internship or equivalent experience and a qualifying examination. Continuing education is required to maintain R.D. status. This certification process encourages high standards of performance to protect the health, safety, and welfare of the public.

To find a registered dietitian (R.D.), the expert in diet, health, and nutrition, ask your physician, call your local hospital, state, or district dietetic association, or contact The American Dietetic Association, 216 W. Jackson Blvd., Chicago, IL 60606-6995; 312-899-0040.

Introduction

We're accustomed to thinking of books as finished products. But cookbooks—especially the one you are holding in your hand—are really midpoints. Recipes begin as ideas; if all goes well, they end as enjoyable, nutritious mouthfuls. The extensive process in between—setting nutritional standards, recipe selection, testing, nutrient analysis, and so on—is aimed at making each recipe tempting to read, healthful to eat, and so tasty you'll want to make it again and again.

RECIPE GUIDELINES

One of the first steps is the development of recipe guidelines—specific nutritional standards to which all recipes will adhere. These were agreed upon jointly by the American Diabetes Association and The American Dietetic Association and are in keeping with the goals of other health organizations such as the American Heart Association and the American Cancer Society, as well as the current guidelines of the United States Departments of Health and Human Services and Agriculture.

The purpose of the guidelines is to facilitate an *overall* healthy diet. Current nutritional goals of the American Diabetes Association include the following: carbohydrate should account for 55 to 60 percent of calories consumed and fat under 30 percent. Protein should make up the remaining percentage. Americans generally need to increase their consumption of complex carbohydrate and fiber and decrease consumption of fat (especially saturated fats), cholesterol, and sodium; most Americans consume more protein than they need.

This does not mean that each *recipe* will have nutrients in the proportions described above but that taken together

1

throughout the days and weeks they make these aims easier to achieve. Unless otherwise noted, the following ingredients are *limited* when they appear in any recipe:

SUGAR: Limited to 1 teaspoon or less of sucrose, honey, molasses per serving.

SODIUM: Limited to 400 milligrams or less per serving.

EGGS: Limited to ½ yolk per serving.

CHOLESTEROL: Limited to less than 300 milligrams per serving.

FAT: Although there is no specific maximum on fat, all recipes are limited in fat and saturated fat.

RECIPE DEVELOPMENT AND TESTING

Where do recipes come from? Recipe "development" is the process by which a recipe is invented or adapted, then refined and tested. A recipe developer always keeps the nutrition guidelines in mind when formulating new recipes, or adapting old recipes to today's standards of taste and nutrition.

Recipe ideas can come from almost anywhere. Some are inspired by the presence of a newly available fresh herb or an unusual fruit or vegetable in the local market. Food magazines or cookbooks provide another source of inspiration, as do the increasing number of "reduced" (in salt, fat, or cholesterol) products that make convenience and nutrition increasingly compatible. (Cooks should read labels carefully, as descriptions may be misleading.) At other times the challenge is to bring an old favorite recipe like fruit cobbler (page 345) up to date.

The recipe developer must plan how many recipes the book will contain and the rough proportion of main dishes, vegetables, salads, soups, and desserts that are wanted. Thought must also go into availability—especially for products like "reduced" items. (Many producers now offer food items with lower salt, fat, and/or sugar content and market them as "lite" or "reduced.") Is an ingredient stocked across the nation? Is it obtainable as easily in Seattle as it is in Tampa or Des Moines? A good recipe developer tests many different brands of, for example, chicken broth, looking for ones with good rich flavor that are also low in sodium and reasonably priced. Moreover, there must be an adequate number of nationally distributed brands before such a product can be included in a recipe. (For example, eleven years ago, when *Family Cookbook Volume I* was published, there were too few "reduced" varieties to assume wide-range availability.)

A recipe cannot even be considered for inclusion unless it has been tested—and retested, and retested. The recipes in this book were tried out first on the developer's family—as good a place as any to gauge appeal to a variety of ages and tastes. They were then retested by a professional tester who made sure they worked the second, third, and fourth time around. Directions may need clarification—Is the turkey cooked or raw? Are apples peeled or not? The tester also judges flavor and appearance. All dishes should be a feast for the eyes as well as the palate. Some recipes are modified, some discarded at this stage.

NUTRIENT ANALYSIS

While the recipe developer keeps the nutrition guidelines always in mind, recipes are put through more rigorous examination during the nutrient analysis stage. It is at this stage that per-portion nutrient content is determined and Exchange values are calculated.

While the calculations can be done manually, a computer can do them much faster. The first step in this process is to ensure that the computer has on file a "nutritional profile" of every ingredient in every recipe. Not a small task since ingredients range from hominy grits and nutmeg to cilantro and reduced-cholesterol Monterey Jack cheese, orange liqueur, porcini mushrooms, and so on. Nutrition profiles for any ingredients not already in the computer must be entered.

What kind of information does the profile cover? Quite

a bit. The USDA Food Composition Tables form its base, supplemented by information on many products direct from their manufacturer. Some of this information appears above every recipe in the cookbook.

The software program used to analyze recipes in this cookbook not only provides nutrients per serving but also provides Exchange List approximations at the same time.(*) To do this, the computer also must be told the Exchange values that apply. It must "know" for example, that a Vegetable exchange contains about 5 grams of carbohydrate, 2 grams of protein, and no fat; a Fruit exchange has 15 grams of carbohydrate, and so forth.

To calculate the per-serving nutrient content, a recipe is divided by the number of people it has been planned to serve. Finally, the computer is told, recipe by recipe, which Exchange List categories to consider—so it won't choose an illogical Exchange like Vegetable if the dish is a dessert. Given all this information, the computer begins a sorting and fitting process that ultimately suggests several best-fit possibilities. Almost every Exchange List designation, however, involves some approximation. The nutrition analyst makes the final decision.

IT ALL STARTS WITH SHOPPING

A good part of the work of keeping recipes within the nutrition guidelines mentioned above was done not in the kitchen but in the supermarket, by purchasing ingredients carefully.

Wise food buying is a way to make sure you are eating healthfully. Decisions are made periodically—say, when you shop for milk or meat or canned goods—but you reap the benefits every day. *Routine* purchasing of healthful ingredients means that when you reach for a product in your refrigerator or on your kitchen shelves, it will already be the one best for you. And

(*)Wheeler LA; Wheeler ML, Ours P: Computer selected Exchange Lists approximations for recipes. *J Am. Diet. Assoc.* 85:700–703, 1985.

certainly, the items listed can be used to make recipes in other cookbooks more healthful.

Shop carefully when purchasing products reduced in sodium, fat, or cholesterol. Flavor and price must be considered. If a "reduced" product's taste doesn't meet your expectations, or if it costs more than seems reasonable, ask your supermarket manager if another brand might be stocked. Sometimes, too, a product lower in one nutrient may be higher in another one you are trying to avoid. Some dairy products lower in fat are higher in sodium; or a product lower in sodium may be high in preservatives. There is no hard-and-fast rule in such cases; whether you want to use the product or not depends on how big a part it plays in your diet, its price, flavor, and so on. The important thing is to read the label and to make a decision based on *your* needs. When in doubt, speak to your doctor, registered dietitian, or diabetes educator.

You may wonder what to do if you find a "reduced" product but the recipe hasn't called for it—nonfat yogurt, for example, when the recipe specifies low-fat. Feel free to buy the "reduced" item as long as it is otherwise satisfactory. When you are preparing dishes from previous *Family Cookbooks*, or other cookbooks, substitute "reduced" varieties whenever possible. Doing so may change the nutrient composition slightly, but probably not enough to alter the Exchange List designation.

Listed below are the shopping and preparation rules-of-thumb we followed in buying and cooking for this cookbook.

DAIRY PRODUCTS

We used low-fat dairy products throughout: skim milk, low-fat yogurt, and, whenever possible, reduced-fat cheeses. You can choose skim milk from the dairy case, powdered dry skim milk, or evaporated skim milk diluted according to instructions. When a creamy taste and texture is desired, *undiluted* evaporated skim milk is an excellent choice. It contains far less fat than cream, but offers the same quality and thickening power.

A wide variety of reduced-fat cheeses is available. But

be sure to choose *natural* rather than imitation cheeses, which tend to be high in additives and sodium. (Where low-fat cheese was not specified, it usually means that the varieties we tried were unpleasant tasting or had poor melting qualities.)

OILS AND FATS

Safflower, corn, peanut, olive, and other polyunsaturated or monounsaturated vegetable oils are used in these recipes. Saturated fats were avoided to the extent possible.

Margarines made from mono- and polyunsaturated oils were used in preference to butter. Sodium was calculated with salted margarine because of its wider availability. Unsalted margarines are fine, too; in the small quantities used, the presence or absence of sodium should make little difference to most people.

FLAVORING AGENTS AND CONDIMENTS

Stock your cupboards with as wide a range of flavoring agents as possible. Some of those we used frequently include: garlic and onion powder (not salts), curry powder, coriander, cumin and turmeric, basil, marjoram, tarragon, oregano, cinnamon, nutmeg. Mustards, lemon, lime, fresh coriander (cilantro), chives, and parsley are other mainstays of flavor.

In cooked dishes, small amounts of alcoholic beverages like vermouth, marsala, dry sherry, brandies, and liqueurs add distinctive flavor and contribute minor amounts of alcohol per serving since some of it evaporates when heated. All those listed above keep well even after a bottle has been opened. Red and white wine are good choices when some of the rest of the bottle will be consumed with a meal since once opened they cannot be kept indefinitely. Alcoholic beverages can add an undertone all their own—and the palette ranges from robust and rich to delicate and subtle.

Flavored vinegars and oils are becoming increasingly available. If you think of vinegar as tasting simply "sour," try some of the new varieties or make your own (see page 129). A huge range of vinegars is available—balsamic, herbal, fruit-flavored, red wine, and white wine. A drop on the tongue will waken your taste buds with the piquant zip of raspberry, tarragon, basil, and many more. The trick in using these is to be sparing but let them carry the tone rather than competing with other, stronger flavors. Flavored oils, too, can provide a distinctive background flavor to the dishes you cook.

We used salsa extensively as a flavoring agent. It comes in mild, medium, or hot varieties, and the mild form is bland enough, with no jalapeño pepper flavor, to appeal even to sensitive eaters. Do not omit salsa, however, if it is called for in a recipe, since leaving it out will affect the liquid content.

Generally we used chile sauce in preference to ketchup; it is easy to find in reduced salt and sugar varieties, and has a livelier tomato flavor. We cooked with reduced-calorie mayonnaise and sour cream, reduced-sodium soy sauce and other such products.

Low-sodium chicken or beef broth, either canned and defatted or in cubes also adds general flavor to main dishes and soups. Although less common, lamb stock, fish stock, and vegetable stock can all contribute significant flavor; but remember to degrease before using. A recipe for chicken stock appears on page 118.

MEATS, POULTRY, AND FISH

We selected the leanest cuts, trimmed them of visible fat, and drained fat after cooking. Poultry was skinned and trimmed of visible fat. Fish is generally low in fat anyway, but any visible fat was trimmed before cooking.

VEGETABLES

Whenever possible, we used fresh vegetables in preference to processed ones. Frozen vegetables are generally lower in sodium than canned. In the case of canned tomatoes, which in the depths of winter are often the best-tasting choice, select varieties with no salt added.

YOU'LL WANT TO KNOW

Just above the ingredient list and cooking method for each recipe is the basic nutritional information per serving and information such as yields and serving sizes.

NUTRIENT CONTENT PER SERVING

Nutrient breakdown (and abbreviations) for the following are listed:

> Calories (CAL)
> Protein (PRO)
> Fat
> Carbohydrate (CHO)
> Sodium (Na)
> Potassium (K)
> Fiber
> Cholesterol (Chol)

Where two choices are offered or optional ingredients listed (for example, "egg substitute or egg" or "optional ½ teaspoon salt"), nutrients for *both* alternatives are supplied.

YIELDS

Yields are generally for four, a good quantity for the average family and an amount easily halved or doubled. Dishes that freeze well and are easier to make in quantity, as with some desserts, have been provided with larger yields.

1 ◇ THE AMERICAN TRADITION

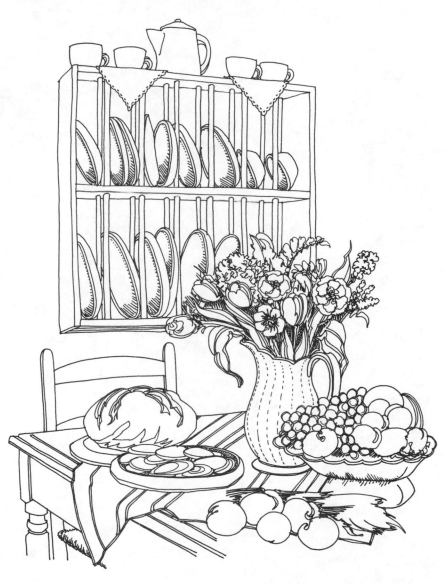

WHAT IS AMERICAN COOKING?

What makes a dish American? Is it native ingredients such as cranberries and corn? Is American eating the meat-and-potatoes cooking of the heartland, or is it the ethnic specialties contributed by the eastern and southern Europeans who flocked to our shores in the nineteenth century or the Latin American and Asian influence current today? Or is American cooking cold cereal, canned soup, and peanut-butter-and-jelly sandwiches?

American cooking in the 1990s draws on all these traditions. It is a cuisine of choice and plenty, of increasing healthfulness and a growing national character.

AS AMERICAN AS . . . ?

It's harder than you may think to label a food as American. Take the hot dog. The frank is really a combination of European tradition and American know-how. It is a German-style sausage dubbed a wiener (i.e., "from Vienna") or a frankfurter ("from Frankfurt") to make it sound more "exotic," and popularized at the 1893 Chicago World's Fair. Cracker Jack, a more truly American product, was introduced at the same fair.

The baked potato took a circuitous route. Native to the Americas, the potato was scorned by colonists, exported to Europe, fancied up by the French—Lyonnaise potatoes, duchesse potatoes—then reintroduced to the United States, where it was prepared with a plainness suited to America—baked in the jacket.

Even Florida orange juice isn't really American. The first orange seeds were brought by the Spanish in the 1500s and planted wherever they went as a protection against scurvy.

How about the apples for American apple pie? Apples go way back, and we grow them well, but they didn't originate here. The Romans grew thirty-six different varieties, some of which Caesar brought to England along with his conquering troops. From England the pilgrims carried apple slips to the New World, and in the early 1800s John Chapman (Johnny Appleseed) traveled 10,000 square miles of the west part of

Connecticut territory—now Ohio—establishing apple nurseries. The first commercial apple tree nursery had been established in Flushing, Long Island, in 1730.

It's safe to say, though, that fresh corn on the cob is an American treat; it originated here and is almost impossible to find elsewhere. Pizza is, of course Italian, but nowhere else will you find it as omnipresent as a snack food. Barbecued ribs is another U.S. specialty. Other than the Chinese, we are the only nation that really likes spareribs, and the barbecue is an American tradition. Others, either unique to these shores or very prevalent here, are fruit mixtures as salads, jellied salads, marshmallows, and soft drinks and milk as beverages.

AMERICAN ATTITUDES

Attitudes toward cooking and eating do as much as ingredients to shape a cooking style. And our attitudes are as distinctively American as turkey.

In other parts of the world, everyday eating is colored by tradition—somewhat as holiday meals are in the United States. Foods are an important part of a person's link to the past; regional traditions, ingredients, and special cooking styles and preferences color almost every meal. The French eat their croissants for breakfast and the Italians, a few miles over the border, eat the hard rolls that are their standard breakfast fare.

We in the United States, on the other hand, have far less respect for tradition. We like newness and variety, and we plunge in wholeheartedly, eating croissants on Monday, bagels on Tuesday, cereal on Wednesday, flapjacks on Thursday, and so forth through the weeks. Our lack of a shared past also shows itself in our penchant for adapting. We take no particular city or region as the ultimate standard in a dish. Chicagoans swear by their thick-crust pizza, New Yorkers by a different dough. Which cranberries are better—Wisconsin's or those of Massachusetts? Idaho or Maine potatoes?

We are confirmed gadgeteers, with a weakness for new devices. Such standard domestic items as the can opener and the paper bag, aluminum foil, plastic wrap, charcoal briquettes, and the automatic toaster were either invented or refined in the United States. Most important, they sold far more briskly here than they did outside this country. Both the stove and refrigerator sold well in the United States, and refinements like the oven heat regulator were eagerly sought.

Americans like small packages—frozen entrées that serve one or two; vegetables for three or four; flour in five-pound bags; breakfast cereals in tiny packages that can be eaten—in the box, if you like—for one only. These can be bought, stored, and eaten at will, with no need to go marketing. In much of the rest of the world, marketing is done every day, as much for social as for practical purposes. Food items are kept in bulk in the market to be sold, with a word or two, a bit of gossip, to the marketer nearly every day.

We ask for contradictory qualities in our eating. We want variety but without too many surprises. We love surefire products like boil-in-bag vegetables, minute rice, cake mixes, canned entrées. We like reliability—garden green beans may taste a bit different each time they are made, but buy a frozen block and you know what you're getting every time. We want foods convenient to prepare, but smacking of home and hearth—"hearty homestyle" canned soups, freeze-dried beef bourguignon.

If other cultures eat from a limited repertoire of foods, prepared in a range of subtle variations, we eat from an infinite variety of foods, and have until recently liked them prepared with virtually no variation at all. We like our food to be reliable—when we open a particular brand of peanut butter, we know that it will taste exactly like the last jar. The same goes for soups, breads, main dishes, and so on. Americans like it that way.

We value convenience and speed: toaster cakes and toaster waffles, instant coffee, butter marked with tablespoon measures, never-fail rice that's ready in a minute, packaged cake mixes, jelly or processed cheese—which, when empty, become juice glasses—canned tuna fish, a glass of milk, square white bread, soft drinks, potato chips and fast food, cold cereal and canned soup, candy bars and chewing gum.

THE LAND OF PLENTY

Red snapper steamed with wild grapes, roast duck stuffed with fruit, deep-fried squash blossoms, maple-smoked turkey, broiled salmon with juniper berries—sound like nouvelle cuisine? These dishes may sound new, but they're Native American specialties enjoyed by the Seminole, Iroquois, Hopi, and Native Americans of the Pacific Northwest.

Native Americans were cooking well long before the colonists arrived. Plants native to the Americas include tomatoes, potatoes, corn, squashes, Jerusalem artichokes, blueberries and cranberries, wild rice, persimmons, chilis, and sassafras. All told, over 2,000 native ingredients were used in Native American cuisine.

Wild fish and game abounded, the turkey and lobster being probably the most well-known. American waters offered crayfish and sea turtles, shad, bass, cod, eel, salmon, trout, bluefish, and bass. On land, there were woodcocks, snipes, partridges and pigeons, rabbit, duck, deer, and buffalo.

A number of edibles did not exist on this continent— apples and oranges, peaches, apricots, and pears were unknown before the colonists arrived. Wheat, barley, rye, and other grains; lettuce, cabbage, lentils, turnips, beets, and carrots; chickens, pigs, sheep, and cows all had to be imported.

THE IMMIGRANT CONTRIBUTION

Between 1607 and the present, more than 45 million immigrants reached the shores of the United States. Our first immigrants, the colonists, established the eating habits of a nation. And they were largely unadventurous ones. The pilgrims were accustomed to English cooking, which is plainer than that of the continent. Their religious beliefs, too, subjugated the beautiful and tasteful to the practical and moral.

For whatever reason, the colonists ate simply, often preferring food that had been laboriously transported from England to the bounty in front of them. Of course there were "pompkin" pies and "cramberry" sauce—both described in Amelia Simmons's *American Cookery*, published in 1796 and considered the first American cookbook. Native American tribes taught the colonists to use cornmeal. So new was the grain to them that practically anything that contained corn was called "Indian" —Indian pudding, Indian cakes (corn bread), and Indian slapjacks (pancakes).

But like the British in India, the colonists tended to try, at least, to recreate Britain abroad. As soon as it was feasible, they imported smaller domesticated animals to dine on—pigs and chickens first, since more could be fit on the crowded ships, then sheep and cows. The British love of sweetness, little use of spices and herbs, and fondness for meat-and-potatoes-type eating spread through New England.

Later immigration took place in waves, influenced by demand for labor in this country; by war, unrest, and famine outside the United States; and in this century by U.S. immigration laws.

Our first 200 years formed our culinary tradition firmly in the mold of simple, hearty eating of a fairly utilitarian nature. From colonial times to the mid-1800s, about two-thirds of our immigrants came from Britain, Germany, and Scandinavia. These immigrants settled along the eastern seaboard, then pushed into the Midwest and northern Midwest.

The later 1800s brought immigrants with markedly different eating habits. The Chinese, who worked on the expanding railroad system and in the Gold Rush, settled on the West Coast. Southern and Eastern nationalities predominated on the East Coast— Italians, Slavs, Poles, Czechs, and others. Many of these new immigrants settled in the cities of New England, the eastern seaboard, and the Midwest, where labor was most in demand. Ethnic neighborhoods developed as families joined relatives and friend joined friend.

Immigrants who settled in cities tended to continue their ethnic eating patterns. Stores had a clientele large enough to stock foreign foods, and the clustering of people of similar tradition tended to allow those traditions to continue. On farms and in rural areas, ethnic people were more scattered, ingredients from the old country more difficult to find, and eating patterns grew more similar to those already established. Many old traditions faded.

In the Eastern European enclaves of Chicago, Cleveland, or New York, vibrant ethnic neighborhoods still exist. Walk into a store and you're walking into a country. European-style produce is sold in bulk—fragrant kegs of dried mushrooms, lekvar by the barrel, strudel doughs, barrels of pickles. In season, you'll find green piles of fresh, water-flecked lettuces, bunches of dill, pots of sour cream, and bunches of fresh green sorrel. Later in the summer, there are the makings of cold fruit soups—sour cherries, plums, or blueberries—to be served as chilly as possible on a hot summer night.

Middle Eastern enclaves on the East or West Coast offer moist, orange dried apricots and barrels of olives—black and glistening, green, cracked, whole, tiny, and shriveled or plump globes. Raisins still on the vine, dates, and figs of varying types all abound, as do breads flat as pancakes and as big as towels.

In the decade between 1900 and 1910, 6 million people arrived, the largest number ever. Progressive tightening of restrictions on immigrants soon followed. From 1927 to 1964, immigration slowed to a trickle, restricted to only 150,000 annually, and strongly weighted in favor of Northern and Western Europeans. Virtually no Chinese or Japanese entered during these years; there was a prohibition on Indians, Indochinese, Afghanistani, Arabs, and so on.

From a culinary perspective, these years were rather barren. Cooking habits, long set in the traditions of Northern and Western Europe, tended to stagnate, with processed foods dominating the national marketplace. In the ethnic neighborhoods of the cities, interesting cooking continued, but for the most part did not spread out into the rest of the country.

A reopening of immigration began with the Hart-Celler Act of 1965, which did away with discriminatory quotas and raised the ceiling on total immigrants. A new wave of immigrants from the Orient, Russia, and Latin America splashed over these shores. It had been half a century since America had seen such a multicultural influx. And this time, unlike the immigrants of the 1800s, whole families, not simply single men, came to America.

Like the immigrants of the late 1800s, these latter-day arrivals tended to settle in the cities—New York, Miami, San Francisco. But today, communications and travel have expanded so much that ethnic eating tends to remain insulated a far shorter time.

FOOD TECHNOLOGY AND "AMERICAN STANDARD" COOKING

From colonial times well into the 1800s, a year-round balanced diet was more the exception than the rule. Many Americans in the late 1700s and early 1800s lived on a diet of salt pork, corn, and beans. Farmers generally ate better than city folks, but even their diets were dependent on the season and the success or failure of crops and livestock.

While home preserving of fruits, vegetables, and meats was common, it was a laborious and chancy affair. Safe preservation of foods, especially vegetables and meats, was a constant battle against molds, enzymes, and bacteria. Woe betide the careless housewife making her weekly examination of canned goods, only to find cloudiness, seepage—or listening with sinking heart to ominous basement explosions.

The late 1800s saw the rapid growth of cities and, with them, the birth of commercial food processing. Although packaged, long-lasting foods had been available before, they were hardly "convenience" foods. Early cans were a far cry from what we know today. An 1824 version was an iron monstrosity weighing more than a pound empty, that had to be opened with a chisel and hammer!

Three pioneers of commercial food processing were Birdseye, Borden, and Kraft. These three men began to shape the industry as we know it today. Clarence Birdseye developed a reliable method for freezing vegetables—a boon both for consumer and producer since it gave the farmer a way of using bumper crops. By 1929, the first Birdseye commercial vegetables were on the market. Although they were slow to gain acceptance, partially because many stores lacked freezing compartments, they grew in popularity. By 1987 American families consumed about 10 million tons of frozen food per year.

As the industry grew and became more regulated, it brought with it for the whole nation the possibility of safer foods and a year-round balanced diet. Later, the industry focused on use of processed foods for convenience and speed. Today home-produced food is for most people more a hobby—or a budget stretcher—than a necessity.

The heyday of processed foods were the years in which whole menus were constructed from processed foods—canned tuna, canned mushroom soup, and potato chips on top. In some recipes, jars or cans were used as units of measurement—one bottle of ketchup and two cans of baked beans, one can of tuna fish—or mushrooms or soup. Sometimes we used packaged foods so routinely that we forgot why. Is a packaged biscuit mix—an American innovation credited to the Shakers—really faster than making them from scratch? Are frozen beans that much faster than fresh?

In the United States, regional and ethnic cooking has had to compete for nearly a century with the thriving commercial foods industry, which is often able to provide at least one or two kinds of a vegetable or fruit on a reliable year-round basis. The tradeoff is often variety so that we begin to think that apples come in only one or two varieties—those that, as it happens, may be bred for shippability and storability more than for flavor.

A supermarket may be selling only two apple varieties—MacIntosh and Red Delicious—in an autumn when local apple trees are bearing Jonathans, Cortlands, Staymans, Northern Spys, Rhode Island Greenings, and Newtown Pippins, each with its special color from burnished copper to dull or brilliant red, yellow, wine-colored, stripy, and flavors in a rainbow variety of tart, sweet, tender or crisp, tart-sweet, spicy or mild, nearly scentless or temptingly aromatic.

OUR TASTES BEGIN TO CHANGE

Recently, ethnic and regional foods—cooking customs, spices, and whole dishes—are becoming increasingly popular. The "mainstreaming" of ethnic and regional specialties has many roots. Among them are our new generations of immigrants. The ease of air travel since the early 1950s allows Americans to taste for themselves the ethnic specialties of Europe, Asia, Mexico, and South America. World War II probably played a role by introducing American GIs to a new world of tastes and brought back with them a taste for wines, herbs, and spice mixtures. The "health food" movement of the past couple of decades also made a contribution.

Another contributor, odd though it may seem, is the processed-food industry itself, which has vigorously marketed Americanized versions of foods previously limited to ethnic communities. Canned or frozen versions of burritos, tacos, pizza, goulash, and blintzes can be found in nearly any supermarket. Dishes like beef bourguignon, Chinese beef with peapods, chicken glazed with fruit, and vegetable medleys introduced us to new foods and food combinations—flat Italian green beans, chickpeas, sweet red peppers, okra, and hundreds, if not thousands, of others. Boxed pilafs showed us that rice wasn't just white and boiled with water.

Admittedly, packaged ethnics often didn't resemble the originals. Sometimes they weren't even particularly tasty, often being prepared with too much salt and sugar. On the other hand, these foods had real advantages—they were ethnic specialties that could be sampled without special shopping and cooking know-how. And they helped introduce a culinarily conservative people to more varied eating.

Today, processed foods are moving into their proper place. We are less likely to overrely on them and more likely to give them a fair try—we use them rather than letting them use us. Canned tomatoes make an excellent pasta sauce; but in August, we're tending more and more to try a fresh sauce, perhaps with an unusual variety purchased from a local farm market. We're more likely to give a little thought to whether it is really more time-consuming to make biscuits from scratch than from a mix. The same goes for dozens of other dishes. Is a frozen pie really easier than a fresh fruit dessert with quick crumb topping? We're not so quick to assume that processed foods are quicker. Sometimes they are, sometimes not.

COOKBOOKS

Cookbooks have always been best-sellers in the United States. And for good reason. We need advice. From the first American cookbook, Amelia Simmons's 1796 *American Cookery*, to the most modern volume showing how to cook Sri Lankan style or with peanut butter, or with exotic vegetables, Americans are big cookbook buyers. We probably buy twice as many cookbooks as, for example, the French, a nation of cooks.

Simmons's cookbook boasted itself as being "adapted to this country and all grades of life"—it was democratic—and Simmons described herself as "An American Orphan." Culinarily speaking, many early Americans were "orphans" in that they could not simply follow the traditions set down by parents and grandparents.

Instead, they had to improvise and adapt, making do without familiar ingredients and figuring out how to substitute new ones. Naturally, whenever possible they pooled information. Many informal cookbooks developed out of women's social clubs and church groups, synagogues, schools, and so forth. Whenever Americans come together, they are likely to pool favorite recipes into a cookbook.

This hunger for information made us avid cookbook buyers. Over the years, we have seen *Fifteen cent dinners for families of six*, an 1877 book, followed in 1889 by *How to Provide a Good Dinner for Four Persons for One Dollar*. A 1904 volume was devoted entirely to oranges—*One Hundred and Twelve Ways of Preparing, Cooking, and Serving Oranges in a Dainty and Appetizing Manner*. . . .

In the late eighteenth century, cookbooks—really compendiums of the most wide-ranging advice—were outsold only by the Bible. Books like *Common Sense in the Farmhouse; Or Young Mother's Assistant and The Queen of the Household: A Guide to the Accomplishments of the Home Work in All Its Various Departments* helped the frontier housewife, many miles from the nearest neighbor, to manage on her own.

One of the best known of these cookbooks was *Buckeye Cookery and Practical Housekeeping*. A midwestern product, *Buckeye* was first published in Marysville, Ohio, in 1876, and grew up as a collection of recipes collected from American women. It contained recipes for bread and cake making, canning, preparation of meats, choosing flour, preserves and pickles, poultry, soups, vegetables, game, fish, and even ice cream and jelly.

It also advised the housewife on marketing, curing meats, housecleaning, and the care of the sick. *Buckeye* includes advice on how to keep pails from shrinking, how to rid the house of rats, how to treat a rattlesnake or dog bite or swallowed glass, what kind of wood—ash—is best for cake baking, how to treat asthma in canary birds, and what to do if you discover your house is on fire.

As democratic as Amelia Simmons, *Buckeye* advised, "Skill in cooking is as readily shown in a baked potato or a johnny-cake as in a canvass-back duck." As a final indication of how seriously the homemaker's job was taken, *Buckeye* reminds its readers, "Bad dinners go hand in hand with total depravity."

Although *Buckeye*'s instructions seem casual to us today— "Dissolve a lump of soda the size of a bean in a spoon of milk . . ." or "To an egg, add a quantity of fine flour to make a nice dough . . ."—they seem to have caused no problem for its readers. Exact timing and measurement did not become fashionable until the twentieth century.

Today, cookbooks are selling as briskly as ever. And thanks to air travel, the telephone, TV and radio, newspapers and magazines, cooking information is being spread continentwide faster and faster. This couldn't have happened 100 years ago, when letters between housewives and cookbooks were the main trade routes of culinary information.

Television is now broadening our cooking repertory. It is an excellent teacher of cooking styles, a sort of electronic grandmother, showing us how to cook Chinese, French, or Italian. We don't have to have watched our Italian grandmother knead flour and egg to just the right consistency, then cut and hang pasta out to dry to create a presentable spaghetti. And each television cook conveys not only information about cooking but a love of food and respect for preparing it well that can be conveyed fully only "in person."

2 ◇ THE REGIONAL STAMP

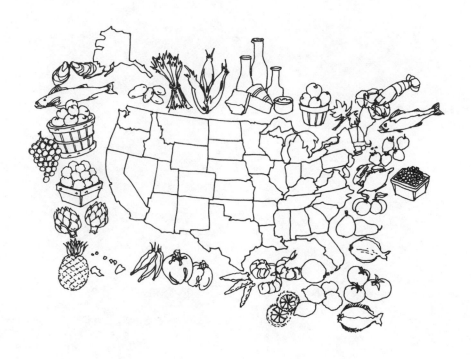

Regional dishes in other parts of the world are based on specific local ingredients—local produce and game, wild herbs and plants. They usually have a centuries-long history, having been passed from generation to generation, and they tend to color everyday dishes. In Italy, for example, there is less an Italian cuisine than a Ligurian, a Roman, a Sicilian, an Emilian—all distinctively different. People tended to stay put, developing and refining a cooking style, then passing it on to their children and grandchildren.

These regional cuisines developed out of long acquaintance, over generations, with the seasons and the climates—it was a cuisine that made use of a limited range of ingredients and foodstuffs, and it did it superbly. American eating starts from a different premise. We want to use everything—we want key lime pie in Minnesota, clambakes in Ohio, and Alaska king crab in Vermont.

Reading a book about regional cooking, a Midwesterner may never have heard of, much less tasted, some "midwestern specialty"—persimmon pie, for example.

Some regional specialties are so well-known as to be clichés. Boston baked beans, midwestern corn on the cob, Texas barbecue, southern fried chicken are all well-known and often well prepared outside their region of origin. Other special dishes are somewhat less popular—Kansas corn chowder, midwestern persimmon pie, St. Louis angel food cake, or Chicago planked whitefish. A third group may not be known at all outside the small town or village where it was developed—locally made cheeses, for example—or because a food does not ship well—cloudberries—or is not particularly in demand outside the area—alligator meat.

In general our regionalism has been more diluted than that of Europe or Asia. For one thing, our regions are bigger and less well-defined, with less of a common past. We also tend to share what we know rather than jealously guard secrets. Recipes for enchiladas and gazpacho can be found in cookbooks of the 1800s.

Finally, we are a mobile people. Historical events like the Civil War and the Dust Bowl have meant huge movements of people from North to South and from East to West. But even as individuals, we tend to be restless. Every year, about one in five American families moves to a different part of the country. As we criss-cross the continent, moving with jobs and marriages, we bring along our regional dishes. A household in which southern corn bread is eaten with salmon of the Northwest coast, or Italian pasta with German cucumber salad—and almost every U.S. family has some such combination—shows the influence of migration.

NEW ENGLAND

Of all regions of the United States, the cuisine of New England is probably best known. The natural products of the area are celebrated throughout the world, as well as the United States—Maine lobsters, Vermont maple syrup, and cranberries.

The classics of New England cooking—New England boiled dinner, codfish cakes, red flannel hash, clam chowder—take us back to colonial days. Beach plum jelly and maple syrup added sweetness. Light cakes are not New England specialties. There were no stoves in early New England capable of maintaining the even temperatures needed for a good risen cake. So hearty pies and fruit cobblers took the day—a good choice, too, because the heavy sugar content helped reduce bacteria and let them be kept longer.

Of course, the coast of New England offered a whole harvest of shellfish and saltwater fish, although the early colonists did not appreciate *Homarus americanus*—America's celebrated lobster. They let these crustaceans pile up on the beaches—two feet high, according to some accounts—ignoring them for what they saw as a greater delicacy—eels.

The influence of the sea extended beyond its bounty of fish. The port cities of Boston, New Bedford, and others were open to the influence of the great sailing ships bringing spices, herbs, and cooking styles from the East. The trading ships that had docked in Bombay brought a taste for curried dishes and spicy condiments. This influence tended to stay in the cities rather than spreading throughout New England. Portuguese cooking, mainly centered around New Bedford, includes sardines, a spicy sausage called linguica, broad beans, and salt cod prepared in all manner of ways.

Despite a generally conservative style and difficult New England growing conditions, by 1796, when America's earliest cookbook was published—in Hartford, Connecticut—New Englanders were using a wider variety of foods than we might imagine. These included melons, artichokes, radishes, cucumbers and lettuces, yams, parsnips, onions, turkeys, salmon, perch, flounder, bass, and cod. Garlic, however, was not used as a flavoring agent: "Though used by the French, [garlic is] better adapted to the uses of medicine than cokery."

Colonists grew beans, both fresh and for keeping, cabbages, herbs, and fruit trees. For flavoring, they employed ginger, almonds, rose water, oranges, orange water, lemons, cinnamon, and nutmeg.

Favorite desserts were English—custards, tarts, gingerbread, and pound cake. Preserves included strawberries and gooseberries, plums and peaches. Just about everything was pickled—as a method of preserving—meat and fish, cucumbers and melons.

THE MIDDLE ATLANTIC STATES

The Middle Atlantic states—New York, New Jersey, Pennsylvania, Delaware, and Maryland—made up the early heart of what has become the Northeast coast megalopolis, an urban corridor that extends in a pattern of cities and suburbs from Boston down to Atlanta. From the very beginning, the Middle Atlantic states were a mix of rich farm country and bustling cities.

Also settled relatively early, the Middle Atlantic states greeted the settlers with a gentler climate and richer growing conditions, allowing all the vegetables and fruits of England to flourish. People of this area, especially the coastal area, did not have to make do with corn, cranberries, salt pork, salt cod, and corned beef. The Garden State, New Jersey, is justly famed for its tomatoes; New York State offers grapes, potatoes, and apples; crabs and poultry come from coastal Maryland and Delaware; the rich farms of Pennsylvania were our nation's first "breadbasket."

New York City typifies the major port cities of the East Coast. It has been the point of entry for the British, Germans, and Dutch, the French, Swedes, and Scandinavians. Italians, Poles, Czechs, Slavs, Russians, and Jews came from eastern and southern Europe. Recent liberalization of immigration regulations has brought Koreans, Indians, Vietnamese, and Haitians. So many people have passed through, or stayed, that the British-Dutch origins of New York have been almost forgotten in the proliferation of new ethnic groups. Currently New York City is home to more than 100 different nationalities, with more than 1.5 million foreign-born people.

Today, New York is a mosaic of ethnic communities, and ethnic neighborhoods do more than anything to keep cooking traditions alive. Little Italy and Chinatown are long established; newer communities are Russian, Indian, and Middle Eastern. There are Greek communities in Queens, Armenians in the Bronx, and Russians in Brooklyn. While the first Chinese immigrants came mainly from Canton and set up restaurants specializing in Cantonese cooking, more recent newcomers hail from other provinces and have brought a whole host of new cuisines, from Szechuan to Hunan and Mandarin.

Little India offers an exotic array of edibles all sold in quantities unknown in the average supermarket: pint containers of mustard seeds, cumin, and coriander; knobs of fresh ginger with the bulk of a fist or dried whole, ground, preserved, or glazed; green and brown cardamom seeds and exotic preserves; mango and coconut milk, pickles and chutneys; tamarind; pistachios by the bushel. Chinatown's wealth includes fresh water chestnuts, live carp, and long, slender string beans, along with winter melons, lychees, and noodles. Filipino neighborhoods have unusual items such as goat meat, guavas, pomegranates, and star fruit. Vegetables include hyacinth beans, snow peas, watercress, nettles, and cashew nut leaves.

The Pennsylvania Dutch—actually Germans ("Deutsch"

is the German word for "German") who came over at the beginning of the 1700s—gave a tradition of hearty eating to the Middle Atlantic states. If the Puritans viewed food chiefly as a necessity, the Pennsylvania Dutch saw it as God's gift for labor. The kitchen was the biggest room in the house and eating was viewed as important.

German specialties like egg noodles, sauerkraut, sausages, and apple butter moved into American cuisine, as well as cinnamon buns, pretzels, and dumplings. The Pennsylvania Dutch used herbs and spices like saffron, coriander, and sage. The favorite meat of the Pennsylvania Dutch was pork, and they used every part of the pig in one way or another—from the muzzle and ears to the feet. Any leftover scraps are combined into the famous Pennsylvania Dutch "scrapple."

Pennsylvania Dutch food was hearty and seasoned with more sophistication than was New England food. The tradition of "seven sweets and seven sours" at each meal gave Pennsylvania Dutch cooking a broad range of flavors. The Pennsylvania Dutch table was loaded down with sweet jams, jellies, and preserves and gooseberries, blackberries, and strawberries. On the sour side, there were bread-and-butter pickles, pickled beets, Jerusalem artichokes, and melon rind, and pickled green tomatoes put up late in autumn so as not to waste the frost-nipped green tomatoes that hadn't time to ripen.

THE SOUTH

From West Virginia to Florida, from North Carolina to Arkansas and Louisiana, the South has always had a tradition of good eating, both plain and fancy. More than any other region, the South can be divided into different subregions, each with its distinctive cooking style.

The area around New Orleans owes its cooking style to both French and Spanish influences, cultures that valued elegance and refinement in eating. In New Orleans, one can sample beignets—light, sugar-powdered snacks—and a huge range of crawfish, crabs, and oysters. Paella, jambalaya, gumbo, and red beans and rice probably owe something to the Spanish influence between 1762 and 1803. Probably more important than the foods themselves is the attitudes toward eating—New Orleans takes its eating seriously.

Florida, too, was influenced by the Spanish, as well as by the tropical ingredients that are found in such profusion here: mangoes, citrus, coconuts. Conch chowder and stone crabs are other local favorites. The latest group of immigrants to exert an influence on Florida cooking is the Cubans, who tend to live in cities and enjoy favorites such as black beans and rice and a savory beef stew known as alcaporado perked up with olives and raisins.

The cuisine of other southern states offers grits, corn bread, and Virginia ham; oysters and pecans, freshwater shrimp, and blackeyed peas. Iced tea and buttermilk are drunk here more than in other parts of the country. Other southern dishes are catfish, hush puppies, spoon bread, and perlow—a rice dish probably related to pilaf.

Good eating in the South goes way back. Virginian Thomas Jefferson, in his 1782 *Notes on Virginia*, describes the fruitful farms of Virginia, producing wheat, rye, barley, oats, and buckwheat. In Virginia gardens, vegetables like parsnips and peanuts, carrots and turnips grew, and the gardens yielded muskmelons, watermelons, okra, pomegranates, apricots, almonds, and plums. In his own garden, Jefferson grew white potatoes and tomatoes—then believed to be poisonous—and experimented with many other plants. He even made his own ice cream!

Greens are a southern favorite, often cooked with salt pork and hot peppers. These may be either cultivated—kale, collard, mustard, and spinach, for example—or simply picked in the wild—dandelion, milkweed, and dockweed.

Plantation cooking was done on two levels—that of the slaves and that of the slave owners. Slaves ate greens, salted pork, and pork variety cuts, as well as small game and freshwater fish. Corn products included hominy and grits as well as hoe cakes—corn bread cooked on the back of a hoe over an open fire. Simple fruit cobblers or sweet potato pone—sweet potatoes, molasses, eggs, shortening, milk, and cinnamon—was a favorite dessert. The slave owners ate better cuts of meat, more fancy cakes and desserts, and generally more labor-intensive dishes, including baked goods like biscuits, yeast breads, and cakes.

THE MIDWEST AND THE GREAT PLAINS

For better or worse, the Midwest defines American cooking in the eyes of many foreigners. And unfortunately, the Midwest has an undeservedly poor reputation as a place of uninteresting eating.

From Ohio to Nebraska, from Oklahoma to Minnesota, change comes slowly to the Midwest, making its way in from the East or West Coasts. But more than any other region it has shaped our ideas about cooking and eating. Midwestern cooking is the solid center point of American cooking, embodying many of the attitudes that make American eating unique—a fondness for large, stomach-filling meals, large portion sizes, especially of meat; desserts of cakes, pies, or cookies rather than fruit or no dessert at all; and a preference for little seasoning except salt and sugar.

Midwestern cooking was influenced by the farm, both its plenty and the labor it took to run it. Midwesterners are engulfed in good food—dairy products in Wisconsin and square miles of wheat, corn, and oats; potatoes, rye, and barley in the north, cattle and hogs in the central and eastern Midwest. Although plenty sometimes leads to innovation, it is want that is more likely to do so, and midwestern cooking has always been plain and plentiful.

Thanks go to the Midwest for the world's fairs. The 1893 Chicago World's Fair introduced a snack called Cracker Jacks and popularized a hot dog on a roll with mustard, in addition to demonstrating, far ahead of its general adoption, the first electric kitchen. Sometime later, in 1904, the St. Louis World's Fair gave the country another portable meal—the hamburger on a bun—and the ice cream cone—first called the "World's Fair Cornucopia," later shortened to cone.

Midwestern eating today is largely "American standard"

cooking, with heavy dependence on prepared foods. Of course, the Midwest has its specialties: corn on the cob, Minnesota wild rice, Scandinavian fruit soups, local cheeses, and Kansas beef.

Pockets of Central and Eastern Europeans—Poles, Hungarians, Czechs, and Slovaks—emigrated to the United States during the late nineteenth and early twentieth centuries. In Chicago, Buffalo, and Cleveland, specialties like Hungarian tailor's collar soup, sour egg soup, cold raspberry or apple soup can be found, as well as poppyseed cakes and sweet and meat-filled strudels.

THE MOUNTAIN STATES

Mountain eating tells of mountain history. Mining brought easterners to the Mountain states—Montana, Idaho, Wyoming, Utah, Nevada, and Colorado—in the late 1800s. The majority of these early miners were single men for whom cooking and eating was more a necessity than a pleasure. Mountain fare reflects this. It was wild fare fit for hunters and fishermen, and for simple preparation often over an open fire.

Although today agriculture is as important as mining once was, many of the culinary high points of the Mountain states are in its wilderness. Montana, for example, produces wheat, beef, and barley, poultry, pigs, and potatoes. But hunting for deer, antelope, duck, and pheasant is popular still, as is fishing for the salmon and trout that abound in its waters.

Basque sheepherders have been driving sheep on the open range since the 1830s. A shepherd is on the move, camping each night and carrying as little as possible—his tent and sleeping roll, water, wine, food, and Dutch ovens. He eats simply but well—perhaps a stew of meat and beans, some garlic for flavor, along with peppers and perhaps some potatoes. The mountains themselves offered meals—small game or brook trout, berries, and perhaps some wild greens or watercress. Mutton jerky can be used for soup, and for bread perhaps some sourdough, that portable loaf for which starter can be carried for years.

The Mormons of Utah, who populate yet another rugged, largely waterless Mountain state, have firm, settled family traditions quite different from the miners and sheepherders that settled much of the rest of the Rockies. When the Mormons settled Utah they did so not to dig mines but to dig the soil. Unlike the largely single men who mined, hunted, and tended sheep, the Mormons settled as families. They are well-known for their excellent preserving and baking.

THE SOUTHWEST

The rest of the United States can thank the Southwest twice over for its cuisine. First, this region was the great corridor for foods whose native habitat was South America—tomatoes, corn, beans, and other vegetables naturally suited to a warm climate. The first Thanksgiving would have been without its corn and squash had not the Southwest passed them on north.

A second thanks is more current, for the Southwest cooking influence is reaching again north and east, introducing timid palates to the bite of peppers, the hearty goodness of beans, and the clash of cool and hot, smooth and rough, light and stomach-filling that characterizes the cuisine of the Southwest. More than most other regions of the United States, southwestern cooking tradition influences daily cooking in the average home.

Texas, New Mexico, and Arizona are noted for those delicious stuffed dishes like the the tamale, burrito, and taco, for chili rellenos and enchiladas. A whole host of tropical fruits and vegetables cools and refreshes southwestern cooking—avocados, plantains, cilantro, the tomatillo, and sapote.

As much as southwestern cooking has its own character, it is in fact a blend of several different cooking traditions that made their way from South America up into the Southwest, having Caribbean and European as well as Native American and Spanish influences.

Some of the cooking traditions that made their way up to the Southwest through Central America are more sophisticated than one might imagine. While some Native Americans prepared and ate simple dishes of corn, beans, and squashes, the Aztec culinary repertory included, in addition to tortillas and chilis, turkey, duck, quail, and lobster. Over a thousand different dishes are recorded. Perhaps the most celebrated gift of the Aztecs was chocolate, from the beans of the cacao tree. The Aztecs used it to make a bitter drink called *chocolatl* from corn flour, herbs, spices, and the cocoa bean. Today, the same bitter chocolate adds depth and richness to chicken mole, a poultry dish that contains chocolate.

The barbecue—a southwestern specialty with nearly any meat available—is one gift of the Southwest to the rest of the nation. More than most other peoples of the world, we like to eat outdoors. Is this a carryover from our Native American teachers who cooked over pits of coals? Or perhaps an inheritance from covered wagon days? Whatever its origin, we seem to like to eat under the open sky with a barbecue, clambake, or picnic. Originally, barbecues were communal affairs, but the charcoal briquette and our penchant for doing things individually led to the backyard barbecue, sometimes with a single family.

Chili seems almost quintessentially southwestern, and it comes in such a host of variations it's hard to know what "authentic" chili is—though virtually every cook claims to make it. A sort of chili con carne—chili peppers with meat—had its place in Native American cooking of the Southwest. But what is the correct, real authentic version of the dish? Beans or not, and if so, which kind, pinto or kidney? What meat, if any—fresh pork, salt pork, veal, and/or beef? Sausage? Stone-ground cornmeal to thicken? Tomatoes? Red wine? Green peppers? Onions? Peanut butter? Oregano, cumin, bay leaf—or just chili? Midwestern versions add pasta, some modern ones outbalance beans and meat with crisp vegetables—celery, carrots, corn. Hot or not? Beer? Mineral water? About the only common ingredient— though not universal—is chili peppers. And chili powder . . . was developed in Texas in 1902 by a German!

THE WEST COAST—CALIFORNIA AND THE PACIFIC NORTHWEST

As much as any group of states, California, Washington, and Oregon have spearheaded a new trend in American cooking based on respect for local ingredients, a willingness to experiment, and a concern for the healthfulness of what is served.

West Coast cooking has always been graced with a variety of the freshest local ingredients from the farm, the orchard, and the sea. The waters of the West Coast are warmer than their counterparts on the Atlantic Ocean; salmon, oysters, clams, and crabs are available year round, for the most part, in profusion. In coastal areas of the Pacific Northwest, plentiful rainfall makes the climate ideal for berries, while the drier climate inland is conducive to the growth of fruit trees such as apples and pears. Oranges and artichokes, avocados, carrots, asparagus, grapes, and lettuce are only a small part of California's produce. The state leads the nation in production of dozens of fruits and vegetables. The wines of California, too, are famed, competing now with the best wines of the rest of the world.

Over the past two decades, California has developed more and more dishes that are not merely fresh but new and interesting. California pioneered new combinations like fish fillet with lemon grass purée; braised cabbage with fresh herbs and Chardonnay wine; wild mushrooms with ginger sauce. Even California sushi—crabmeat with avocado—is a typically California dish.

The eclectic, experimental nature of the Western seaboard can't be accounted for easily. California's great tradition of wine growing may have sensitized many palates; and the winegrowers themselves, largely French and Italian, come from food-loving cultures to begin with. California's rich ethnic mix of cultures living side by side in a land of plenty adds another ingredient. California cooking is Asian in its respect for freshness and attention to appearance. The Middle East adds another typical set of ingredients—eggplants and chick-peas, lentils, beans and olives and dates, yogurt, and sweets of honey and nuts. A fondness exists for lamb, often cooked over an open fire on skewers.

The health movement found a home in California, a state whose climate allowed year-round outdoor activity. These influences combine to shape a cuisine that is eclectic and selective, valuing simplicity and freshness but with a use of materials that seems to delight in finding new combinations rather than sticking with old ones well prepared.

The influence of West Coast cooking can be found in many newer recipes, which often specify ingredients with a precision that would have been thought unnecessary previously. Current recipes take into consideration a huge variety of tastes and textures, which tends to spread this awareness to the cook, the eater, the shopkeeper, and so on. A recipe may specify balsamic or hazelnut vinegar, for example. Mustard is not simply a yellow sauce for hot dogs, but can be made with tarragon or other herbs, smooth or grainy, bitingly sharp or sweet. Of the thousand or so varieties of rice, today's cooks are looking for the rice that best fits their needs—nutty, textured brown rice; Italian arborio in a creamy risotto; or any of dozens of others.

ALASKA AND HAWAII

Alaska and Hawaii hold somewhat the place in American cooking today that the Southwest did in the 1800s. Only a few mainlanders have sampled Hawaiian poi or Alaskan reindeer steaks, though we've probably heard of both. These two states have yet to make their major contribution to U.S. cooking styles. Hawaii, of course, is a major source of tropical fruits like pineapples and a chief producer of sugar cane, supplying sugar to the rest of the United States. Native Hawaiians originally lived almost exclusively on fish and fruit, using coconut milk for almost every purpose that cow's milk is used elsewhere.

Beginning before 1820, trading vessels, then planes, brought people of many other cultures to Hawaii. To the original Polynesian islands, the Yankees brought pigs, chickens, and goats, as well as canned meats. Soy sauce and the hibachi came with the Japanese, while Koreans added pickled products like kimchi. A doughnutlike sweet called malassadas came with the Portuguese.

Today, Hawaiian traditions include the luau, a bountiful feast with its barbecued meats, poi—a paste made from the taro root, and plentiful fresh tropical fruits. Other foods more plentiful in Hawaii than in most of the mainland include macadamia nuts, coconuts, pineapple, and papayas, fruits that so much of Hawaii's rich volcanic soil produces in its fertile farmland.

Alaska is a state of extremes that remains as mysterious to us as the colonies were to England so many years ago. Winters in Alaska can mean wind-chill factors of 100 below zero, but brief summers may be hot and plagued with mosquitos. Alaska contains the tallest mountains and the longest coastline. Alaska's Matanuska Valley produces giant-size vegetables— cabbages weighing over fifty pounds and rhubarb taller than a five-year-old child. But most of Alaska contains too little rather than too much plant life; in many places, mosses and berries are the only plant life around.

Even better from a hunter's or fisher's point of view, the fish may be as big and plentiful—and therefore as easy to catch—as those described by first visitors to the continent. They are so numerous because they inhabit streams deep in the wilderness, where the rod and reel are rarely seen.

Alaskan cuisine today is built mainly around two sources: food imported from the lower forty-eight and wild foods, meat, and fish. The state has plentiful caribou, ducks, moose, and reindeer, as well as bear and, from Alaskan waters, salmon, trout, and crab.

THE NEW REGIONALISM

The current rebirth of interest in food, flavors, and subtlety has coincided with increased interest in health and less time to prepare foods. Less reliance on salt and sugar opened our palates to a whole range of other flavors drowned out by oversalting and oversugaring.

We have returned to earlier cooking—that of the Native Americans, for example, using many of the thousands of ingredients they employed. In 1877, the *Buckeye* cookbook suggested a sophisticated salad of cultivated and wild greens, including lettuce and chicory, dandelion greens, asparagus, and watercress. Farm markets are making this sort of a salad a real possibility again, and this time for city and suburban dwellers, not only for rural people.

There is a new interest in wild foods like mushrooms, fiddlehead ferns, and berries. Some, like sorrel and purslane, are actually garden escapees originally imported from Europe but which jumped the fence and established themselves as wild in previous centuries. Neglected for years, while Americans narrowed their tastes to a few mild-tasting lettuces, they are now being rediscovered. Farm markets are finding eager buyers for perishable, rare, and difficult-to-grow varieties of fruits and vegetables.

Only a few years ago, the most elegant restaurants of any region of the United States tended to have as specialties French dishes—escargots, filet mignon, vegetables sauced in the French style, and desserts too. The best cooks in a region, then, weren't cooking regionally but all served versions of the same—continental—cusine. Often results were poor. Filet of sole meunière served with old fish could please no one.

Today the menu is more likely dictated by freshness and availability. Squash blossoms or banana flowers will only be served when they meet certain standards. The same goes for autumn venison or quail in Vermont, Dover sole and caviar anyplace. Michigan filet of pickerel and Oregon wild mushrooms may be combined into a succulent dish, but only when both are up to standard.

The new regionalism has two distinct strains—the experimental and the puristic. Some cooks look for new and different combinations from around the world. Mixtas from Guatemala clearly reflects its native American, Spanish, and German origins—a tortilla with guacamole topped with sausage and sauerkraut! The California roll, a type of sushi, does the same, combining crabmeat and avocado in a Japanese preparation.

Other examples are coriander pesto, mint or basil sherbets, Philippine spicy shrimp with cucumber sauce, chickpea spread with pickled lime, poached salmon with ginger sauce.

Another trend in regional cooking is represented by the cook who will use only local ingredients—a New England cook who won't use California raspberries or Georgia peaches. He or she waits until full summer when native crops ripen and will try to find as many different local varieties as possible. Why? Regional pride is one reason. Another may be the attempt to know thoroughly local ingredients and encourage their growth. And a purely human motivation, perhaps, is that anticipation adds a spice all its own.

3 ◇ EATING AND HEALTH: TRENDS IN AMERICA

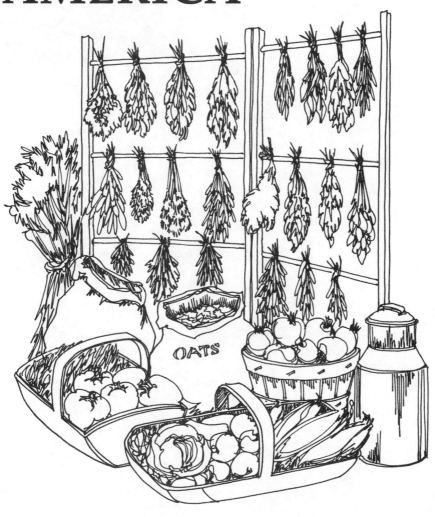

Are you a member of the Clean Plate Club? The idea that it is of utmost importance to eat every scrap of food on the plate to avoid waste has been a guiding principle of American family eating through much of the twentieth century. And it is an idea that has probably, especially in a land of such plenty, contributed to overeating and obesity.

Its origins are pure Pennsylvania Dutch. One Pennsylvania Dutch saying expressed the idea with perfect, if horrifyingly graphic, economy: "Better a burst stomach than wasted food." An interesting contrast to American attitudes is that of Chinese parents, who teach their children to leave the table when they are 70 percent full. They also plan meals so that fat, vegetable, fruit, and meat or fish together make up only about one-fifth of the calories consumed; four-fifths is a grain such as rice.

In a land of plenty, ideas guide our eating as much as the available foods. Beliefs about desirable meal size and composition directly affect the amount we eat and our food choices. Over the years, different trends in eating have dominated. But generally Americans are a "bigger is better" people who favor meat over any other nutrient.

EATING ON THE FARM

As late as 100 years ago, three-quarters of Americans lived in rural areas, and rural eating in a land of plenty tended to make us believe that big meals were good meals. The strenuous physical exercise that was essential to farm life demanded large meals. In wintertime, large meals helped the farmer keep warm in houses that lacked central heating.

Bills of fare suggested in the 1877 *Buckeye Cookery* were in such proportions that it is hard to conceive of today. They must have demanded extraordinary labor, time, and planning.

Some typical suggested meals:

BREAKFAST: Oatmeal mush, veal cutlets, fried liver,

fricasseed potatoes, new onions; toast, hot pocketbooks [a sort of spongy turnover served without a filling for breakfast or tea]; asparagus, radishes, coffee, and chocolate.

OR

Blackberry mush, beefsteak, snipe on toast, sliced tomatoes, stewed corn, applesauce, warm rolls, coffee, tea, or chocolate.

DINNER: Gumbo soup, roast lamb, mint sauce; fried chicken, peas, string beans, potatoes, cucumbers, lettuce, radishes, ripe currant pie, bohemian cream, strawberries, lady's fingers, rolled jelly cake, coffee.

OR

Tomato soup, baked beef with Yorkshire pudding, chicken pie with oysters, mashed potatoes, hominy, dried corn and lima beans, cream slaw, celery, bottled cucumbers, fig pudding with lemon sauce, apple pie, apples, figs and nuts, coffee and tea.

SUPPER: Cold lamb, cucumber salad, bread, strawberry shortcake with sweetened cream, gooseberry fool, tea.

OR

Cold beef, chili sauce, lobster salad, warm French rolls, peach shortcake, delicate cake, iced milk and iced tea.

A meal we might recognize as more familiar was what *Buckeye* termed "An economical dinner"—boiled beef, lima beans, boiled potatoes, squash, sliced tomatoes, apple tapioca pudding.

CITY EATING

For the rich, city meals in the last century could be just as tremendous, even though people needed far less energy for city living. City meals were much richer than their country counterparts, with delicacies and wines imported from Europe. Home entertainment and restaurants featured a stong French accent, with cream sauces, truffles, petits fours, mayonnaises, and pâtés.

For the poor, good nourishment was often hard to find. Inadequate sanitation was a major hurdle. Tenements lacked toilets, baths, and running water. Garbage dumped into central airshafts accumulated window-high.

Meats were not infrequently spoiled. Fear of fresh fruits and vegetables compounded the problem. Diseases such as cholera were thought to be transmitted by raw fruits and vegetables, so people would not eat them even when they were available. This belief continued until well after World War I. Fresh milk presented another problem. Well into the 1930s, milk was kept refrigerated at local shops and was obtained daily. The shopkeeper would dip into the refrigerated can, and transfer a few ladlesful into a smaller, home-size can, which would be carried along the street, often without a lid or covering, sometimes in sweltering weather, home for breakfast.

A BETTER WAY

Was there a healthier way to eat? As you munch on a graham cracker or eat a bowl of cold cereal, you may not realize it but you're squarely in the middle of an early American health food movement. The trend toward eating less meat, more fresh vegetables, fruits, and complex carbohydrates didn't start a decade ago but more than a century ago. And the trend has been coming and going ever since.

Interestingly, in the United States healthful eating has been associated as much with the pulpit as with the palate. A number of food reformers have been preachers eager to convert others to a better way to eat.

The Reverend Sylvester Graham was one of these. Graham crackers have become so much a part of standard American fare that it may be hard to realize that there was a reverend, after whom graham flour (a finely ground, whole wheat flour) was named. A man of the cloth who held strong views on eating, Graham stressed the need to eat a variety of foods. Going against medical opinion of the 1830s, Graham believed that the diet should be high in fresh fruits and vegetables, preferably eaten raw.

As you might expect, he advocated whole wheat products —graham bread, graham muffins, graham pancakes, and graham gems—a muffinlike preparation. So much did Graham's thinking take hold that you can find graham flour recipes in nearly every cookbook written after Graham's time.

Somewhat later in the century, just after the Civil War, another set of dietary reformers with religious underpinnings were the brothers Kellogg. Both brothers were Seventh Day Adventists, a religious sect that advocated meat once a day only and otherwise plain living—abstinence from salt, alcohol, smoking, and spices.

Dr. J. H. Kellogg, a physician, and his brother ran a sanitarium in Battle Creek, Michigan, that, along with dozens of cures for all manner of ailments, served its clients a cold breakfast cereal first called Granola, then Granose. It was developed as a healthy alternative to the hearty quail-on-toast, fried oysters, Saratoga (potato) chips, and pancakes type of breakfast so common at that time.

A patient of his, Charles Post, developed another dry breakfast cereal, first called Elijah's Manna, then Grape Nuts. This was followed by Post Toasties. Kellogg's countered with Corn Flakes. . . . And the battle was on. Americans loved the new, easy-to-prepare, and apparently healthful dry cereals.

Another religious group that has influenced American eating habits in a positive direction is the Shakers. During the eighteenth and nineteenth centuries, the Shakers ate generally healthily, well, and interestingly. They made great use of herbs, using rosemary to season spinach, for example, and cooking ham in cider. They preferred their vegetables cooked only briefly and used the cooking liquid as a base for other sauces and gravies. The Shakers were American, too, in their general practicality and inventiveness. They sold herbs in packets—along with recipe ideas for using them—and vigorously marketed jams, pickles, and preserves. Their major culinary innovation, still used today, was a premixed pancake preparation containing flour, baking soda, salt, and shortening.

TOWARD A SCIENCE OF NUTRITION

People have been thinking about the healthfulness of what they were eating long before there was any science of nutrition. Sometimes they stumbled across important nutritional facts or developed them by trial and error over the centuries. At other times, food beliefs were erroneous.

Vegetables and fruits have gone through extended periods of being feared. Often they were believed to transmit disease—or, like the potato and tomato, to be poisonous. One 1837 cookbook advised cooking green beans 1½ hours to "improve" the vegetables' taste and to make them "more healthful." (It is not surprising that these recipes also described exactly how to delicately pick up the vegetables so they would not fall apart!) Once the value of vitamins and minerals was appreciated, some hundred years later, shorter cooking times became the rule.

Meat, too, has gone through various trends. Miss Beecher's 1846 cookbook warns, "The most injurious food of any in common use is the *animal* oils and articles cooked with them . . .", a remarkably accurate view by today's standards. In the first part of the twentieth century, housewives were advised to eat meat sparingly and *never* to feed it to babies. But by 1959, meat had come to possess near-supernatural qualities: "*Protein* is the magic word," one cookbook author writes enthusiastically. She fondly describes a child with its "little, greasy face and . . . equally greasy fingers" begging for more lamb chops. Today's mother, seeing the same vision, could only think of tiny, greasy coronary arteries.

The science of nutrition is in fact a fairly new one. Until

recently, very little was known about the nutritional value of foods; a common nineteenth-century belief was that although foods looked different, they were all essentially the same. The modern idea of nutrition—that for health human beings must take in certain quantitities of a variety of nutrients—is less than 200 years old.

In some cases, ethnic eating, refined over the years, resulted in a nutritionally adequate diet. The understanding that vitamin C prevents scurvy was not known explicitly until the 1930s; nevertheless, Native Americans generally avoided the disease by consuming spruce tea, which is rich in vitamin C, or eating berries; their pemmican always contained dried berries rich in vitamins.

Pellagra is another vitamin-deficiency disease that did not occur among Native American people but did among westerners who did not combine foods in the traditional way. Pellagra was common in the South in the early 1900s among poor people whose major source of food is corn; it occurred infrequently in the Southwest because the lime used in Mexican tortillas makes the niacin in corn available for nutritional purposes.

The scientific study of nutrition can be thought of in three major periods, the third of which we are just entering. During the 1800s, foods were first classified into types—carbohydrate, fat, and protein—though they were not called by these names. It was also realized that the energy the body uses is related in some way to the amount of food consumed and how active the body is.

During the first half of the 1900s, amino acids, vitamins, fatty acids, and minerals were identified and recognized to be essential in the human diet. In the 1960s trace elements were also given their important place in the diet.

The third period began in the second half of this century, and required almost a reversal of thinking: Nutrition science began to focus not on deficiencies but on the effect of eating habits on chronic degenerative diseases like cancer, diabetes, and diseases of the heart and blood vessels.

4 ◇ AMERICA'S LIFE-STYLE . . . AMERICA'S HEALTH

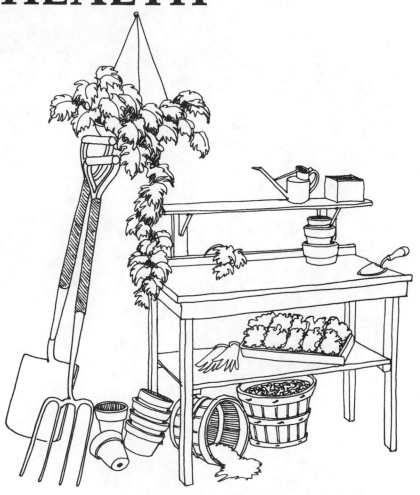

Medical progress over the last century has meant longer lives for Americans, as well as others throughout the world. Disease prevention through vaccines for polio, diphtheria, whooping cough, measles, and others greatly reduced or eliminated the occurrence of these diseases. The 1930s' development of antibiotics like penicillin virtually halved the number of deaths from infectious diseases like pneumonia and tuberculosis; with development of more antibiotics, this number has steadily declined since the 1940s, dramatically lessening the danger of infectious diseases.

Life expectancy has climbed steadily for both men and women since records have been kept. In 1850, life expectancy at birth was only about thirty-eight years; by 1900, the figure was forty-eight; by 1940–51, sixty-six; and by 1982 we could expect to live to be seventy-one years old. Do we deserve a pat on the back for this achievement? Certainly. But this is far from the best we can do.

While we've added over 30 years *from birth*, the gain is much smaller as a person grows older. In 1850, a 50-year-old could look forward to living to be 71½ years old; in 1982, a 50-year-old could expect to live to 75½—only four years longer. Why the small difference? Because many of the diseases that have been eliminated or nearly eliminated affect younger people; also, the conquest of infectious diseases, which affect people of all ages, means that someone who would have died of an infection at 12 or 30 now lives many years longer.

At the turn of the century, there were about 68 cancer deaths per 100,000 people; in 1983, this figure had risen to 188.3 per 100,000. During the same period, heart disease rose from 153 per 100,000 to 327.6 per 100,000. Many of the diseases that are now shortening our lives are ones that tend to strike middle-aged or older people—diseases that, when we were living a shorter time, we didn't have a chance to develop. In addition to heart disease and cancer, other common illnesses include high blood pressure, strokes, diabetes, and atherosclerosis.

But aren't many of these "natural" to growing old? Increasing evidence suggests that the answer is no. A growing consensus of health organizations over the past several decades points the finger at life-style. Factors such as what we eat and drink, how active we are, and whether or not we smoke cigarettes may all help to determine whether and when we develop such long-term chronic diseases. Better news still, modifying such risk factors may enable us to prevent or postpone poor health for many years.

There are similarities among many of the diseases that are affecting Americans today: They occur in older people and they are influenced by life-style. A third important similarity is that many of them are interrelated. Polio and measles are separate, distinct diseases. In contrast, diabetes and heart disease, or stroke and high blood pressure, or obesity and diabetes are interrelated. People with diabetes are more prone to heart disease, for example, and high blood pressure increases the risk of stroke. This is important to keep in mind because if we develop one of these diseases we may be increasing our risk for some others. In preventing or controlling one we are bettering our chances with others.

THE ROLE OF NUTRITION

The 1988 *Surgeon General's Report on Nutrition and Health* took a hard, careful look at the role of nutrition in the long-term chronic diseases that are prevalent in the United States today. Their findings show that diet plays a crucial role in a number of conditions. More important, in almost all cases, THE SAME CHANGES IN DIET CAN LESSEN RISK FOR A BROAD NUMBER OF DISEASES.

In addition, the major chronic diseases, including diabetes, are treated with a generally similar nutrition plan. In other words, you should be eating in much the same way if:

+ You have diabetes or it "runs in the family"
+ Your blood pressure is borderline high
+ You have had a heart attack or stroke

♦ You are worried about cancer
♦ You are in excellent health and want to stay that way

Diet appears to play a part in at least five major diseases: heart disease, cancer, stroke, diabetes mellitus, and atherosclerosis. Overconsumption of alcohol contributes to three others: automobile accidents, suicide, and chronic liver disease.

Several decades ago, dietary recommendations of the major health organizations differed significantly from one another. Now there is general agreement among the recommendations. The American Diabetes Association, The American Dietetic Association, the American Heart Association (1985), the National Cancer Institute Guidelines (1988), the American Cancer Society (1985), and the USDA/DHHS Dietary Guidelines for Americans (1985) agree on almost all dietary issues.

Although each association words its recommendations slightly differently, they speak with one voice: Cut down on fat and sugar, increase fiber, eat several servings a day of fruits and vegetables, avoid being overweight; if you drink alcohol, do so in moderation; limit salt intake. Guidelines of the National Cancer Institute also recommend limiting salt-cured, salt-pickled, and smoked foods.

As a best estimate, 30 percent of cancer deaths are attributable to tobacco and 35 percent to diet. Among the dietary components that appear to be related to various types of cancer are the following: Breast, colon, and prostate cancer are related to increased intake of fat and calories and increased body weight. [Increased alcohol intake is associated with increased cancer risk as well.] A diet high in smoked, salted, and pickled foods is linked to cancers of the stomach and esophagus.

Interestingly, studies have also found that some foods are protective. Increased intake is associated with decreased rates of cancer. High consumption of fruits and vegetables is linked with decreased cancer of the lung, breast, colon, prostate, bladder, mouth, stomach, and cervix. A high fiber intake is associated with decreased colon cancer.

Type II diabetes—also known as "adult-onset" or

"maturity-onset" diabetes, which makes up about 90 percent of cases of diabetes, is strongly linked to obesity. At least 80 percent of persons with type II diabetes are overweight, and weight loss remains the best treatment for this kind of diabetes. (For more about diabetes, see Chapters 5 and 6.)

The role of diet in cardiovascular disease—diseases of the heart and blood vessels—is well established. Studies over several decades have linked it to high levels of saturated fats, total fats, and cholesterol consumption.

High blood pressure, too, has a dietary component. Sodium, alcohol, and overweight all tend to increase blood pressure. If you have high blood pressure and eat a lot of salt or drink a lot of alcohol or are overweight, reducing any of these is likely to help you reduce blood pressure. It has been suggested that normalizing weight would normalize blood pressure in nearly 50 percent of white people and nearly 30 percent of blacks.

Some success has already been achieved in response to the growing information available over the past decades. Deaths from coronary heart disease are decreasing, a fact that experts attribute to both better medical care such as improved ability to treat people having a heart attack and to changes we have already made in our eating and activity habits. Between 1964 and 1985, the age-adjusted death rate from coronary heart disease has decreased by more than 42 percent; one study shows that 30 percent of the decline is due to reductions in plasma cholesterol.

Today more people know what high blood pressure is, and that it endangers their health, than was true in the 1960s. Almost every adult in the United States has had his or her blood pressure measured at least once, and nearly 75 percent have had blood pressure checked within 6 months. Compared to the early 1970s, twice the number of people with high blood pressure have it under control through treatments such as weight reduction and salt and alcohol restriction.

Although not everyone who is obese develops poor health, overweight increases the risk for a host of diseases, among them gallstones, sleep apnea, and osteoarthritis. Illness from heart disease, cancer, diabetes, digestive diseases, and cardiovascular disease is associated with extreme overweight. Although the causal link has not been pinned down precisely, the numbers speak clearly.

In addition to these diseases, dietary excess or imbalance play a role in a number of other problems that may shorten life (especially by interacting with other diseases) or make it more costly or uncomfortable. These include osteoporosis, tooth and gum, and bowel disease. Osteoporosis, for example, causes over a million bone fractures a year in people over forty-five. It is estimated that by age ninety, one-third of women and one-sixth of men will have fractured a hip. Between 12 and 20 percent of these will die; many others will have to live in nursing homes. Diseases of the teeth and gums may contribute to inadequate nutrition, especially in older people.

HOW WE'RE EATING NOW

The main conclusion of the *Surgeon General's Report* is: "Overconsumption of certain dietary components is now a major concern for Americans. While many food factors are involved, chief among them is the disproportionate consumption of foods high in fats, often at the expense of foods high in complex carbohydrates and fiber that may be more conducive to health."

According to the Report we are eating too much:

Fat. Americans are consuming 34–37 percent of calories as fat, versus the 30 percent that is recommended. Moreover, of that amount, 40 percent was saturated, 40 percent monounsaturated, and 20 percent polyunsaturated.

Cholesterol. Men are consuming 435 mg/day; women, 304 mg/day; and children, 254 mg/day. Recommended amounts are under 300 mg/day.

Protein. Women are consuming 144 percent of the recommended daily allowance (RDA) of protein, men 175 percent, and children a whopping 222 percent.

Sodium. For men and children, estimated mean intakes of sodium—not counting table salt—were more than the maximum upper safe limit; for women they were within that limit.

We are eating too little:

Fiber. We consume from 10 (children) to 18 (men) grams of dietary fiber per day, compared to the 20–35 grams recommended by The American Dietetic Association and the maximum of 40 grams recommended by the American Diabetes Association.

Calcium. Women get only 78 percent of the RDA, while men get 115 percent.

Iron. Women, 61 percent and children, 88 percent of the RDA; men, 159 percent.

Vitamin B_6. Women, under 70 percent and men, under 90 percent of the RDA.

Folacin. Women, under 60 percent and men, under 90 percent of the RDA.

Zinc. Women, under 70 percent of the RDA and men, 94 percent.

Copper. All groups are below the RDA.

Magnesium. Women, 72 percent of the RDA and men, 94 percent.

Carbohydrates. we consume 45–52 percent of total calories from carbohydrate. The American Diabetes Association and The American Dietetic Association recommend 55–60 percent, with all or nearly all complex carbohydrates and the type of natural sugars found in milk and fruits. The Report noted our low consumption of complex carbohydrates and fiber.

We are eating about the right amount of: Vitamin A, vitamin E, vitamin C, thiamin, riboflavin, niacin, and vitamin B_{12}.

Although one would think that use of nutrient supplements might rectify the problem relatively easily, the Report found that supplements are likely to be used by the people who are least likely to need them. People who took vitamin pills were those who tended to eat an otherwise healthy diet, one especially high in fruits and vegetables. And of course, overconsumption of supplements can be dangerous; some supplement users take up to sixty times the RDA of some nutrients.

WE'VE MADE A START

Even though we are not eating as well as we might be, changes in buying trends indicate an increasing concern with following the recommendations of various health organizations. The Report notes the following trends, based on yearly per capita availability (as a measure of consumption) or various foods, compared to the years 1965–67.

- We are eating less meat, more poultry, and somewhat more fish. Consumption of meat has declined from 123.6 lbs to 120.9 lbs, while poultry has increased from 30.6 lbs to 47.6 lbs. Fish and shellfish consumption has increased somewhat from 10.8 to 13.8 lbs per person.
- Egg consumption has declined from 40 to less than 33 eggs.
- Low-fat milk and milk products have skyrocketed from 41.7 to 111.4 lbs. We are eating more of all kinds of cheeses, from 9.8 to 21.5 lbs.
- We are eating more fats, but less saturated fats and more vegetable fats. Butter and lard consumption have declined from nearly 17 to 13.5 lbs. Meanwhile, total vegetable fat, like margarine and salad oils, has increased from 35.2 to 50.6 lbs.
- We eat more fresh fruits (52.1 vs. 62.1 lbs) and vegetables (62.6 vs. 79.7 lbs).

♦ We eat virtually the same amount of beans, peas, and nuts—14.8 lbs then and 14.6 now.
♦ Total use of caloric sweeteners has increased from 114.8 lbs—already high—to 127.1 lbs per year.

Food labeling has helped the consumer make more educated food choices—although many people still need help deciphering them. And over the past decade, the food industry has become more responsive to the consumer's demand for healthier food choices. Oat bran, for example, was introduced in the form of muffins, cereals, and so forth soon after its beneficial effects were publicized. Too, many products are marked prominently as being free of tropical oils. Soup and salad bars have proliferated, expanding the availability of fresh foods.

ACTIVITY

If nutrition can help us to live a long and vigorous life, another component in healthy living is keeping active. We've made progress in that area, too.

Many more of us are making exercise a part of our lives than were in the 1960s. In addition, we tend to expect more of ourselves. Exercise recommendations of thirty years ago often stopped at forty-five—with the implicit assumption that those over that age could not or would not be pursuing exercise. Today there are eighty-year-olds who are running marathons. We realize that exercise, sensibly pursued and individualized, should continue as long as possible.

We are also exercising more sensibly. If we have health problems or if we are middle-aged, we are likely to seek medical advice before plunging into vigorous activity. A complete physical examination is a wise precaution for anyone trying to keep fit. And physicians today are more likely to encourage their patients to exercise and to know how to tailor a program to the fitness and interest level of the individual.

5 ◇ TOWARD THE TWENTY-FIRST CENTURY

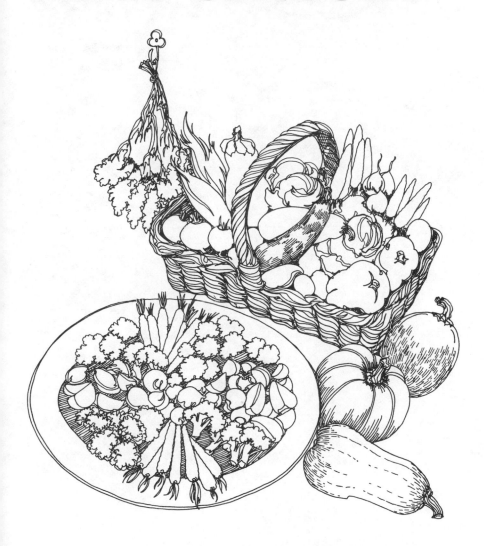

WE'VE DONE IT BEFORE

The U.S. government has been recommending nutritional modification to its people since 1917. These recommendations have changed over the years, though, as scientific knowledge increased and as the habits of the American people changed. For example, the 1917 guidelines stressed the importance of eating a variety of foods, including those with starch and fiber. Its other two recommendations might surprise people of today: to be sure to include sugar and fat in the diet. There were no recommendations at this time in regard to maintaining ideal body weight or limiting cholesterol, salt, or alcohol. It was not until 1979 that these recommendations came on the scene.

Past national campaigns to change U.S. eating habits have met with some success. National attention was focused on nutrition around the time of the First World War, when many draftees had to be rejected because of nutrition-related illnesses.

The first nationwide food fortification was begun a few years later, when iodine was added to salt to prevent goiter. In the forties, wheat flour was enriched with iron, thiamin, niacin, and riboflavin and vitamin D was added to milk, to allow the calcium it contained to be used by the body. Programs such as these helped to nearly eliminate, by the 1950s, diseases such as rickets (caused by lack of vitamin D), pellagra (caused by lack of niacin), night blindness (caused by lack of vitamin A), and other deficiency diseases.

MODERATION AND VARIETY: INGREDIENTS FOR A HEALTHY DIET

The Surgeon General's Report on Nutrition and Health was published in 1988. One of its purposes was to examine changes the American public might make that would reduce the risks for chronic disease such as coronary heart disease, stroke, cancer, and diabetes.

The Report made a number of recommendations for the U.S. population:

EAT A VARIETY OF FOODS

If there had to be one single message conveyed and adopted from the Report, it would probably be: Eat a variety of foods.

Varied eating has been part of every set of government recommendations since 1917. Why? Each food group has its own special strengths and weaknesses, some we may not even know about. Trace elements (substances that occur in infinitesimally small amounts in foodstuffs) have only in the last few years been identified and recognized to play a crucial role in major body functions. Because the science of nutrition is as yet so young, there is more to be discovered. Vitamin pills—valuable as they are for some—contain only the vitamins and minerals that are already *known to be* necessary to the diet. The ideal way of obtaining all the nutrients you need remains a varied diet.

Varied eating is interesting eating. Given some time and reasonably educated tastebuds, processed foods, though some are quite nutritious, begin to taste the same—they're made that way. To put real zing on your plate, you'll find that doing it yourself is the way to go, with our ever-increasing selection of fruits and vegetables.

MAINTAIN DESIRABLE WEIGHT

Interestingly, obesity was rare as a medical condition until relatively recently. There were, of course, isolated instances of very overweight people, but in England it was only in the eighteenth and nineteenth centuries that it began to be found in the upper classes—not coincidentally, since it was during this time that machines began to do more and more work formerly done by people. A more sedentary life-style had begun.

Scientific investigation of obesity, which had gradually become more widespread, was spurred by the publication in 1940 of "Adipose Tissue: A Neglected Subject." The first time that information on life expectancy was linked to weight was in 1913, followed in 1940 when the Metropolitan Life Insurance company published tables of desirable weights. It became clear that overweight people were more inclined to develop diabetes, cardiovascular disease, and other illnesses.

Animals tend to overeat if they have available to them tasty foods, especially those high in fat and sugar and low in fiber—foods similar to those we see in our supermarkets every day. Because such foods tend to be especially tempting, high in calories, and low in vitamins, minerals, and fiber, they should be kept to a minimum in the diet.

Eating fewer calories than the body needs to function or increasing activity beyond the calories ingested is the only way to lose weight. Try to become accustomed to leaving the table before you feel "stuffed." It is probably no coincidence that the Chinese and Japanese, with their low-fat cooking, also prefer to leave the table not quite full.

AVOID TOO MUCH FAT, SATURATED FAT, AND CHOLESTEROL

Major sources of fat in our diet are high-fat cuts of meat, cold cuts, gravies, and salad dressings. Saturated fats are generally solid at room temperature; major sources are fats from animal products—butter and cream, fat of poultry and meat, and egg yolks.

Steer clear of too much fat by choosing foods low in fat, such as vegetables and fruits, lean meats, fish, and poultry and looking for low-fat milks and cheeses. Learn about food preparation methods that keep fat to a minimum—stir-frying or oven baking instead of deep-frying, for example.

In selecting packaged and processed foods, read the label; avoid animal fats and tropical oils like palm and coconut which are also saturated. Some snack foods, packaged entrées and side dishes, and desserts contain lots of fat. As the food industry realizes that this is a concern of many Americans, your task should become easier.

EAT FOOD WITH ADEQUATE STARCH AND FIBER

A 1985 study found that the leading sources of calories in the U.S. diet are the following: [G. Block et al, *Am J. Epidemiology*, 1985]: White bread, rolls, crackers, doughnuts, cookies, cakes, alcoholic beverages, whole milk, hamburgers, cheeseburgers, beef steaks, roasts, soft drinks, hot dogs, ham, lunch meat, eggs, french fries, and potato chips.

The absence of fruits and vegetables, whole grains, dried legumes is striking—even given the fact that most are relatively low in calories. All these are excellent sources of complex carbohydrates and fiber.

AVOID TOO MUCH SUGAR AND TOO MUCH SODIUM

In addition to the sugar bowl and the salt shaker, both sugar and sodium are found in many processed foods, snacks, desserts such as cakes and pies, and sugared breakfast cereals. We are one of the few peoples who seem to prefer sugar and salt together. Either can be found alone, of course. Chips, salted nuts, cold cuts, and lunch meats all contain lots of salt. Candy, many desserts, and caloric soft drinks have lots of sugar.

If you are trying to cut down on sugar and salt, remember that less sugar and salt may make food taste better. Test yourself. Take a few bites of some fruit you especially like—a mellow peach, a fragrant honeydew melon, a crisp sweet-tart apple. Notice the special mix of flavors that makes you like it. Next, take a couple of swallows of a cola drink—regular or diet will do—then another bite of fruit. Without doubt, the strong sweetness of the drink probably wiped out all the "personality" of the fruit. That's the way with both salt and sugar. Unless used with a very light touch, they are blunderbuss seasonings that tend to erase the uniqueness of what they touch. Using less of them actually allows you to taste more.

IF YOU DRINK ALCOHOLIC BEVERAGES, DO SO IN MODERATION

There is no need to consume any alcohol at all, and drinking in moderation should be okay for most people. But alcohol should be used wisely. Don't drink when you are pregnant, driving a car, or doing anything that requires your good judgment.

WHAT IS DIABETES?

People with diabetes are at more risk for many common nutrition-related diseases. There are two major types of diabetes mellitus. About 7 million Americans have *diagnosed* diabetes mellitus, while another 7 million probably have the disease without knowing it or receiving treatment for it. The main differences in the two types are outlined in the table below. Although type I or insulin-dependent diabetes is better known, type II or non-insulin-dependent diabetes affects many more Americans.

Type I	Type II
Who Gets It?	
Mainly children and young adults	Mainly people who are "over forty and overweight"
Sometimes older people	Blacks, Hispanics, and Native Americans are especially vulnerable
What Goes Wrong?	
The body stops making insulin	The body doesn't use insulin efficiently
Onset	
Usually sudden	Usually gradual
Symptoms	
Frequent urination	Any type I symptom
Extreme thirst and hunger	Vision changes

Symptoms (con'd)

Weight loss

Exhaustion

Nausea and vomiting

Slow-to-heal cuts

Itchy skin

Numbness or tingling in fingers or feet

Treatment

Insulin

Sound nutrition

Consistent eating pattern

Exercise

Weight loss, if overweight

Sound nutrition

Exercise

Sometimes pills

Cause

Not completely known

Viral infection

Immune system malfunction

Not completely known

Family history important

Obesity plays a role

People with diabetes are two to four times as likely to die from heart disease and up to six times as likely to have strokes than those without diabetes. Kidney disease affects 10 percent of people with diabetes, and visual impairment and amputations because of poor circulation also take a toll. All told, while diabetes itself causes about 37,000 deaths per year, it contributes to about four times as many deaths.

NUTRITIONAL GOALS FOR PEOPLE WITH DIABETES

Like the rest of the U.S. population, people with diabetes come in all colors, shapes, and sizes. And people with diabetes usually have the same nutritional needs and the same eating habits as everyone else. Since nutritional excess and imbalance can contribute to many chronic diseases, including some types of diabetes, it is not surprising that the nutritional changes recommended for the majority of the American public are wise for people with diabetes, too.

The three main goals of nutritional management of diabetes are:

- Maintain appropriate blood glucose and blood-fat levels
- Maintain reasonable weight
- Eat a varied, nutritionally adequate diet

How can these goals be achieved? If you aren't familiar with diabetes, you may think that *the* most important task for a person with diabetes is to avoid sugar. In fact, while limiting intake of sugar is wise for people with diabetes, other actions are just as important.

For people with type I diabetes, these goals are best accomplished with the ongoing help of a registered dietitian. Of prime importance in keeping blood glucose levels appropriate is consistent timing of meals and snacks so that they coincide as precisely as possible with the action of injected insulin. Toward the same end, type I people must also try to eat about the same amount of food from day to day. Fat intake should be kept to under 30 percent of daily calories because high blood-fat levels contribute to cardiovascular disease.

Weight control is not a widespread problem for people with type I diabetes, although a regimen too high in insulin may facilitate weight gain and too little insulin may lead to weight loss.

For people with type II diabetes who are overweight, as most are, the top priority is weight loss. Nothing is more important than that, and with weight loss can be expected to come improvements in blood glucose, blood pressure, and blood fats. Limiting fat intake is also a high priority. Of somewhat less importance is limiting sugar intake. For those who take insulin, meal timing and consistency is also important.

Some people with type II diabetes are of normal weight. For them, the single most important priority is consuming limited fat. If they take insulin, meal timing and consistency, and sugar limitation are somewhat less important.

A registered dietitian can help people with any type of diabetes choose wisely, as outlined in the *Surgeon General's Report*. For more information on meal planning, see Chapter 6.

THE CHALLENGES WE FACE

We are more concerned about nutrition and health than we ever were, and yet the present and future makeup of our nation presents some formidable challenges to healthful eating. An aging population is one. Families with two working parents are another; a third is the large number of single people in modern-day America. Each of these groups faces special problems.

AN OLDER AMERICA

In 1900, we were a young nation, with people over sixty-five representing only 4 percent of the population. By the year 2030, it is expected that the over-sixty-five group will make up 21 percent of the population.

What we know about nutrition now can influence how our whole nation will age. The older we become, the more our past behavior affects our present health. In the younger years, chronological age (age in years) and physiological age (our body's overall health) are usually fairly similar. As we age, though, the two may be quite different.

Some seventy-year-olds are physiologically closer to an average eighty-five-year-old—in terms of number of medical problems, ability to see and hear adequately, muscle and joint health, mental alertness, balance, and ability to withstand and recover from injuries such as falls, and illnesses. Other seventy-year-olds feel and act much like people fifteen years younger—active, energetic, their health intact, perhaps playing some sport regularly, and able to be active in hobbies and other social organizations.

Although older Americans need fewer total calories, their need for nutrients, including protein, fat, and carbohydrate and vitamins and minerals, is the same as for other adults. The major nutritional problem faced by elderly citizens is not overnutrition but undernutrition and often an unbalanced diet. Decreases in the senses of smell and taste may make eating less pleasant, decreasing the desire to eat. Poorly fitting dentures may add to the temptation to simply prepare the quickest, easiest meal—sometimes a bowl of cereal three times a day.

Shopping may be an obstacle, with heavy parcels to carry or difficulties with transportation. Even opening cans or jars may be a problem, as may the physical exertion it takes to move about the kitchen carrying pots and pans and the flexibility required to reach higher shelves to assemble all that is needed for a meal. Finally, many older people are lonely and simply find cooking a full meal too much of a bother.

Here are a few tips for older Americans, especially those whose health or vigor is already impaired.

Accept help. Many people want to help an older friend or relative but aren't sure what to do. It's up to the older person to give some guidance. For example, you might ask for a large casserole or a hearty soup, divided into individual portions to be frozen and used as needed. Remember that what might be a single meal for a family can provide many, many meals to an older single person. Avail yourself of community services that will bring prepared meals to your home. Social services sometimes provides these free to some senior citizens; private companies provide the same service for a fee. Devices can help to open cans or bottles.

For protein sources, think beyond meat. Eggs, legumes, dairy products, and peanut butter can supply protein. Canned fish and hard cheese keep well. Both are good protein sources, and hard cheeses can be melted over whole wheat bread for a quick and easy main course.

Some delicatessen counters allow purchase of cooked beef, turkey, and other meats in small quantities. A whole roasted chicken may provide a single person almost a week's worth of protein if leftovers are packaged into individual-size portions, then frozen or refrigerated carefully and rewarmed or eaten cold.

Fresh vegetables and fruits may present real problems. Shopping for them daily is nearly impossible for many older folks, yet buying large quantities is inadvisable since they spoil relatively fast.

If you can market for fresh veggies only once every two

weeks, eat the most perishable first—fresh spinach, tomatoes, or cucumbers; move on to keepers like carrots and celery, then on to the frozen vegetables. Try buying a whole cabbage, eating half gradually for salad and freezing the other half; it can be eaten later, quite soft and pliant, as part of a casserole or stuffed cabbage. Or cook all of the large package of green beans; eat some for dinner and refrigerate the rest, perhaps with a little oil and vinegar—they're a great addition to your salad the next day and will keep well for a week or so.

If your supermarket is one of the growing number with a salad bar or deli counter, and if your budget allows, they are an excellent way to have a restaurant-size variety of fresh fruits and vegetables in the exact quantity you want. But steer clear of salad dressings (you can add your own at home) and prepared salads, both of which add weight to your tray and up the cost.

For fruits, try frozen juices or fruits. And don't forget dried fruits, which keep well and can be cooked briefly in a little water if chewing them is a problem.

WORKING PARENTS

If the problems of older Americans have to do with failing health and loneliness, those of the middle generation are little time, little energy, and divided attention. How, with this hurry and bustle, do you achieve the Surgeon General's advice of nutritional moderation and variety?

A problem typical of many families is lack of variety in the vegetable category. Many families stick to a few tried-and-true veggies—peas, green beans, iceberg lettuce, for example. Use common sense in introducing your family to a wider variety of vegetables. Of course, start gradually. Don't bombard your family with okra, brussels sprouts, and kale all in one week just because you are on a new-vegetable-a-day binge.

You may want to dress up an already familiar dish like carrots—mix cooked carrots with toasted bread crumbs, parsley, or even chopped nuts or a small spoonful of coconut. For the first time, make a small quantity and serve a small quantity.

Be sensitive to texture. If your family likes hearty soups, add a small quantity of a new vegetable to a soup that's already a favorite. Do the same with casseroles and meat loaves—both excellent ways to sneak in a new vegetable or two. Try a quiche with Swiss chard or spinach. Add lentils or brown rice to a meat loaf. You can even add grated zucchini or carrots to breads or cakes.

If your family only likes plain foods, respect their tastes. Serve new sauces on the side, so that only a little at a time can be sampled.

Right now, do a refrigerator/cupboard survey. When you open the fridge door, what is the first thing you see? A half-finished package of bologna? Mayonnaise? Last night's dessert leftovers? In the cupboard, are you faced immediately with a bag of potato chips and salty crackers? Try being a little sneaky. When putting away leftovers, store high-fat or sugary foods in aluminum foil or brown paper so they can't be seen. Or move the mayo to the back row. Up front, place a bowl of fresh vegetables, cut up and ready to be eaten, or one of fresh or dried fruits. The kinds of foods you'd prefer your family to eat can be stored in transparent wrap.

Try making frozen fruit—it's a great treat on a hot summer day. Simply array berries, grapes, mango slices, melon balls, or whatever else appeals to you on a cookie sheet in the freezer. Don't crowd them; let each freeze individually. When fruit is frozen—it takes only an hour or so for small fruits—put them all into a plastic bag and return to the freezer. Fruit will keep well for a week or so, and although its texture will change, it is fine for simply popping into your mouth or even used in place of ice cubes to cool a summer drink.

SINGLES

Younger singles are a busy group. They often block in every minute of the day and the night as well. While some singles are attentive to their health, for others, age and illness seem too far away to worry about. Singles can eat as they wish; there are no family constraints to dictate meal timing or nutrition.

Here are a few tips for singles.

If you like to cook, do so on weekends and freeze in single-serving portions. Or try getting together with friends for dinner at one another's houses once a week. Each person can bring an already prepared dish, or, if there is more time, the whole crowd can cook the meal together.

Prepared and frozen entrées combined with a micro-waved green vegetable and a starchy vegetable can be a balanced meal ready in minutes.

If you eat out, use the doggie bag. Singles probably eat out more than others; be sure to bring home leftovers—some portion sizes are large enough for two meals.

Singles have much more flexibility in eating than family members; this can have both advantages and disadvantages. Sometimes singles neglect full meal preparation and, like older people, stick to one favorite food—tuna sandwiches or pizza, for example. Try to use this flexibility to advantage. Singles can set their own eating hours, eating pretty much when and what they like. Although this practice can be abused, some people find that if they eat only when hungry, and only enough to satisfy hunger, it is easier to maintain their weight.

Look for a supermarket or greengrocer that sells perishables in small quantities; though these may be more expensive, the waste you avoid may make the cost the same as buying larger quantities and having half the package spoil.

Every once in a while, do a nutrition assessment. Think back over the foods you've eaten during the last week or so, then, using the Exchange Lists (see page 361) or other versions of the ADA cookbook, determine the quantities of each nutrient you are taking in. Are you short on fresh fruits and vegetables? Whole grains? Legumes and beans? You may want to consider a vitamin supplement. Try adding the nutrients you're missing to those you ordinarily eat. If you feel you could never get enough pizza, try topping a bought pizza with fresh peppers, onions, zucchini, or broccoli and rewarming it.

ACTIVITY

Human beings are meant to be moving. Although most of us are aware that using a muscle can increase its size—in weight lifting, for example, or bodybuilding—we are often not aware that the body is responsive to lack of physical activity as well.

Take, for example, the case of someone in bed for a month because of a broken leg. As little as one month of complete disuse can cause muscles to shrink to half their normal size. Bone, too, is responsive to use. Without the stimulation of physical activity, even when there is sufficient calcium, vitamin D, and other nutrients, the bones may begin to thin. In both cases, it is the needs of the body, signaled by its *activity level*, that control the health of muscle and bone.

Are you fit? Being in good shape is not simply a matter of how many sit-ups, push-ups, or chin-ups you can do. And you won't find the answer in the exact number of miles you walked or ran last week.

A better—though not perfect—test of fitness is how you feel, especially if you are middle-aged or beyond. Do you have enough energy to handle your daily activities energetically, then, when the day is over, do you have energy to pursue hobbies or other leisure time activities? Are your joints stiff, or do they feel limber and flexible? If you suddenly have to run for a bus or climb several flights of stairs, are you able to take these stresses in stride or do they leave you gasping for breath?

If you feel draggy and lethargic, tired in midafternoon, or exhausted by the end of your work day the culprit is probably inactivity. It's a common belief that activity makes you tired. And of course it is true that day after day of hard physical labor, especially if combined with substandard nutrition—as was common a century or two ago—is exhausting and can be debilitating. But viewing activity as mainly tiring is outmoded thinking.

Far more common today is the person who has an office job for eight hours and eats a full complement of nutrients but lives a sedentary life. In this case, activity would be energizing, adding hours to each day in terms of extra energy, vigor, and simply more enjoyment of what you do.

Exercise has so many other bonuses they are hard to count. In the short term, extra energy is perhaps the biggest payoff. Those with diabetes may also experience improved blood glucose. In the long term, activity tends to prevent osteoporosis and helps to control weight and blood pressure. Exercise is also good psychologically, as well as for bowel function and joint flexibility.

6 ◇ EXCHANGE LISTS FOR MEAL PLANNING: AN EASY WAY TO VARIED EATING

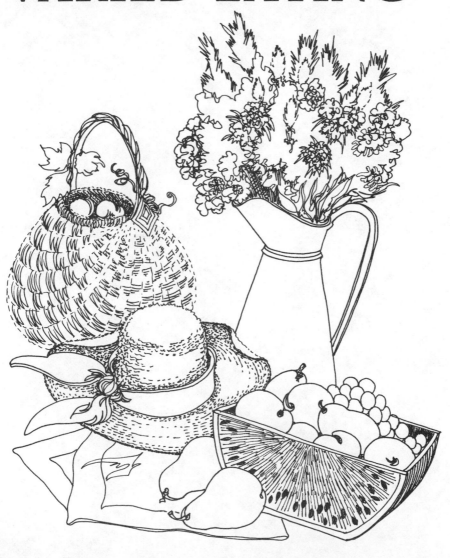

At first glance they may seem intimidating. But their popularity is good evidence that, once you get to know them, Exchange Lists are user-friendly. The *Exchange Lists for Meal Planning* have been published by the American Diabetes Association and The American Dietetic Association for nearly forty years. During that time they have become the most common meal planning systems for people with diabetes, offering a relatively easy way to achieve important goals of therapy.

Although the large majority of people who use the Exchange Lists take insulin, the lists may benefit non–insulin users as well. They may aid in weight loss, for example, by helping individuals achieve the right caloric levels. And the wide range of choices they offer may make sticking to a weight-loss plan easier. In fact, a new version titled *Exchange Lists for Weight Management* was published by The American Dietetic Association and the American Diabetes Association in 1989.

The lists—there are six of them—are simply groupings of nutritionally similar foods. In the specific amounts listed, each food on a list is equivalent, in terms of calories, protein, fat, and carbohydrate, to every other item on that list. For example, on the Starch/Bread List, 1 slice of bread = 3 tablespoons of wheat germ = 8 animal crackers. Any item can be used in place of, that is, exchanged or traded for, any other item on the same list.

Nutritional consistency is an important treatment goal for insulin users: each meal should contain approximately the same proportion of protein, fat, and carbohydrate and the same number of calories as every other meal. Yet to be appetizing—and maximally nutritious—food choices should also be varied. The "trade-offs" on the Exchange Lists offer a means to achieve nutritional similarity while offering a variety of choices.

Monotonous they're not. The Exchange Lists provide plenty of variety. From bagels and water chestnuts to peanut butter and pumpkin seeds, you're likely to find your special favorites. Or you might want to experiment with new foods. If you were to try, one by one, every item in the Starch/Bread List with every fruit on the Fruit List, you'd have 2,784 combinations. At the rate of one taste test a day, you'd need 7½ years to sample them all!

A MEAL PLAN BUILT AROUND YOU

A meal plan is a personalized eating pattern worked out with you by your doctor and registered dietitian. Don't think of it as a diet. If you are of normal weight, it won't be low in calories. And, rather than stressing foods not to eat, it shows you how to eat, combine, and enjoy a large variety of foods. In fact, a good meal plan should actually broaden your eating choices.

Your meal plan will take into account both your nutritional needs and your personal preferences. Your doctor and dietitian will assess your general health and determine the number of calories you'll need based on your sex, age, weight, and life-style. The more energy you expend in growing or exercising, the more calories are allotted. An active eighteen-year-old boy usually needs more calories than a girl the same age. The larger you are, the more calories you'll need to maintain that weight, and women who are pregnant or breast-feeding should consume extra calories. Occupation is another factor: A thirty-five-year-old, 153-pound man who sits at a desk all day may need only half the calories he would if he had an active physical job like construction work, lumbering, or deep-sea diving.

The American Diabetes Association and The American Dietetic Association currently recommend that up to 60 percent of your daily calories come from carbohydrate, less than 30 percent from fat, and the rest from protein. Although adequate for most people, this macronutrient distribution may vary. If blood fats are high (hyperlipidemia), your doctor may recommend a diet with a fat content closer to 20 percent than 30 percent of total calories. And if you have kidney disease, lower protein levels may be advisable. Of course, the calories subtracted from one area must be made up in another. Cutting back on fats, for example, will probably mean eating more carbohydrate.

If you have food allergies or other diseases requiring diet modification, your meal plan must be tailored to avoid one food or another while providing adequate nutrition. And, of course, it must supply the proper amounts of vitamins, minerals, and fiber.

Using this information, plus knowledge about the type

of insulin schedule you are on, the dietitian helps you to map out a meal plan. A common plan is three meals and two or three snacks daily, timed to coincide with peak insulin action. But yours may be different, depending on factors such as your insulin regimen, the rate at which your body absorbs and uses insulin, your life-style, and your preferences. If you're trying to lose weight to control non-insulin-dependent diabetes, just three small meals a day will do nicely.

YOUR PREFERENCES COUNT

The better a meal plan suits you, the more likely you are to follow it. So the dietitian will have *you* in mind as much as nutrition. She or he will take your food preferences into account. If you don't like milk, for example, you dietitian can substitute cheese or yogurt. But if you prefer that even these be minimal in your diet, she or he will suggest alternatives or combinations of other foods that provide the same nutrients but are more palatable to you. Meats, leafy green vegetables, and whole grains can provide much of the protein, calcium, and vitamins that milk would supply in someone else's meal plan.

Although concentrated carbohydrate sources must be restricted, your dietitian can help you work an occasional favorite sugar-containing treat into your meal plan. She or he may suggest that you reduce portion size or modify a recipe, or may help you find a brand that is low in sugar. Ethnic preferences are important, too. To prepare a favorite family dish—Greek *stifatho*, Mexican *menudo*, or Indian *biryani*—your dietitian can provide nutrient information and suggestions in modifying recipes, if necessary.

CHANGING THE MEAL PLAN

Expect your meal plan to change. As a child grows, the meal plan must be modified to include more calories. During adolescence, when the temptation to go along with the crowd is strong, unscheduled snacking is common and fast-food meals with friends occur often. The dietitian can suggest wise fast-food and snacking options. If alcohol use begins, the dietitian along with the physician can explain the rules of safe drinking to the young adult.

Adult meal plans need modification as well. An avid skier may need more calories during the ski season than in the summer months. A promotion from assembly line to supervisor may mean that you're settling a dispute during lunch hour or reviewing safety regulations at snack time. Trying to stick to your former, more regular meal regimen will be difficult, and diabetes control may suffer. Anyone who is in an "emergency" profession will need extra advice. Firefighters or surgical nurses, for example, have such unpredictable schedules that they'll need special help in meal scheduling and dealing with delays.

GETTING TO KNOW THE EXCHANGE LISTS

The Exchange Lists offer an ingenious solution to a complex problem. The problem is this: As an insulin user you need nutritional *sameness*, but as an eater you want *variety*. Nondiabetic people and many people with type II diabetes have the whole day—or several days—to balance out their nutrients. A lunch that's too high in fat can be made up for by eating less fat at dinner. The insulin user doesn't have that luxury.

Constructing a meal that contains the proper proportion of carbohydrate, protein, and fat is difficult indeed. Each food contains a *mixture* of nutrients, in different proportions. Moreover, nutrients vary in the calories they contain. (Carbohydrate and protein have four calories per gram and fat has nine.) By grouping together nutritionally similar foods, the Exchange Lists do most of the calculating for you, allowing you to focus on foods, not grams, calories, and proportions.

Take a look at the Exchange Lists themselves—you'll find them in the Appendix. Notice that foods are grouped into six categories. The six groups are: Starch/Bread; Meat; Vegetable; Fruit; Milk; and Fat.

Most of the foods listed in any particular group will make sense to you. Spinach, lettuce, and green beans, for example, appear in the vegetable group, while hamburger, shrimp, and chicken are grouped with other meats. There may be a few surprises, however. The trick to understanding them is to remember that the groups are based on *nutritional* similarity. Take the avocado, for example. It's green, it grows on a tree, and you'll find it in the produce section of your supermarket. To all appearances, it's a vegetable, but, at nearly 70 percent fat, its nutrient profile is close to that of margarine, mayonnaise, olive oil, and other foods on the fat list. It bears little resemblance to a typical vegetable like asparagus, which contains less than 1 percent fat. Nuts, edible seeds, and nondairy coffee creamer also appear on the fat list because of their high oil content.

All foods in the Starch/Bread List contain 15 grams of carbohydrate, 3 grams of protein, a trace of fat, and 80 calories. Most breads, rolls, and English muffins have this nutritional profile. But so do dried beans, peas, and lentils. Corn, lima beans, and yams fall into this category, too. Nutritionally, these vegetables have more in common with grains than they do with spinach or zucchini. For similar reasons, cheeses, peanut butter, and tofu are found in the Meat and Substitutes List.

FREE FOODS, COMBINATION FOODS, AND FOODS FOR OCCASIONAL USE

Important additions to the *Exchange Lists for Meal Planning* are three new or greatly enlarged categories that allow easy, more flexible use of the lists: Free Foods, Combination Foods, and Foods for Occasional Use.

Free Foods are foods or drinks with fewer than 20 calories per serving. These may be eaten in either unlimited quantities or very freely. You may eat all you like of foods such as spinach; dill pickles; sugar-free hard candy, gum, and gelatin; coffee; tea; and diet sodas. Green peppers, sugar-free jams and jellies, low-calorie salad dressings, and ketchup may be enjoyed two or three times a day in reasonable quantities. Herbs, spices, "lite" soy sauce, and ¼ cup of cooking wine to enhance flavor may also be used liberally.

Average exchange values are listed for Combination Foods like homemade casseroles and macaroni and cheese. Such food mixtures do not fit well into any one Exchange List, although most are prepared in similar enough ways to be classified here. Exchanges for some popular packaged products like chunky soups, spaghetti and meatballs, and sugar-free puddings have also been calculated.

Finally, there's the Foods for Occasional Use section, containing ice cream, granola, cookies, and (uniced) cakes. Most people can enjoy these high-sugar treats in small portions every once in a while, although you'll want to talk to your registered dietitian about the best way to fit them into your meal plan and how frequently you can have them.

HOW EXCHANGE LISTS WORK

When a registered dietitian devises a meal plan with you, several combinations of exchanges, all satisfying your nutritional needs, are available. For example, for a meal containing about 60 grams of carbohydrate, 25 grams of protein, and 16 grams of fat (the approximately 60 percent-10 percent-30 percent distribution), any of the following combinations, plus many more, would be possible. NOTE: This is only a SAMPLE. It is not a meal plan.

CHOICE A: 2 Starch/Bread exchanges
2 Meat (lean)
3 Vegetable
1 Fruit
0 Milk
1 Fat

CHOICE B: 3 Starch/Bread
1 Meat (medium-fat)
0 Vegetable
1 Fruit

> 1 Milk
> 1 Fat
>
> CHOICE C: 2 Starch/Bread
> 0 Meat
> 1 Vegetable
> 0 Fruit
> 2 Milk (low-fat)
> 0 Fat

As you can see, there are many possibilities. Depending on your preferences and nutrient needs, your meal plan might be designed to include many choices from the Starch/Bread List, or the Milk List, or the Vegetable List and fewer from a list whose choices appeal to you less. (In theory, one could even have a meal identical in *macro*nutrients to those above by choosing from only two categories: 3 Low-Fat Milk exchanges and 1½ Fruit exchanges, although such a meal would not provide a wide enough range of micronutrients.)

PRACTICE USING EXCHANGE LISTS

Once you and your registered dietitian have worked out a meal plan, the next step is to "fill in the blanks" with the foods you have chosen. At first this takes some practice. You'll want to be in touch with your dietitian since adjustments to the meal plan are often made as you're getting used to it. At first, it's a good idea to measure portions carefully, both to ensure accuracy and as a way to learn to estimate portions correctly (a skill that's invaluable when you're eating in restaurants).

The Exchange Lists have been designed to use common measures you'll have around the house, such as teaspoons, tablespoons, and cups. Pretzels and french fried potatoes, certain fruits, and pancakes and breadsticks, for example, are measured in inches, so you'll want to be sure you have a ruler. A postage scale or simple balance is good for weighing meat portions. Although all this may sound difficult, getting the feel of a portion size will come easily. Soon you'll be estimating by eye and only referring to rulers and scales as a periodic check on accuracy.

The meal plan designed for you will have a certain number of exchanges from various categories at each meal. For lunch, your meal plan might specify:

2 *S*tarch/Bread
2 *M*eat (lean)
1 *V*egetable
1 *F*ruit
0 *M*ilk
1 *F*at

Using this particular combination of exchanges, you might come up with menus as varied as these:

2 slices bread (2S) in a sandwich with
1 teaspoon of mayonnaise (1F) and
2 ounces of turkey (2M)
½ cup of cooked green beans (1V)
Large green salad (free) and low-calorie dressing (free)
1 apple (1Fr)

OR

1 cup of spaghetti (2S) topped with
¼ cup of cottage cheese (1M) and
2 tablespoons of Parmesan cheese (1M)
Salad of 1 large fresh tomato (1V) with ⅛ avocado, cubed (1F), and low-calorie dressing (free)
½ mango (1 Fr)

OR

1 cup of bean soup (1S, 1V, 1M)
1 ounce of diet cheese (1M)

Large green salad (free) with 1 cup of low-fat croutons (1S) and low-calorie dressing (free)

Raisin-peanut mix (2 tablespoons of raisins, 20 small peanuts: 1 Fr, 1F)

Breakfast? Choices need not be limited to toast and margarine, fruit juice, and coffee. Using the exchanges and some help from a registered dietitian, a person of Japanese background might plan a breakfast of tea, rice, and pickled vegetables; a Swede might choose black bread, cheese, and coffee; or an Italian might prefer Foccacia and caffè latte. You could even get your starch and fat exchanges from chow mein noodles left over from last night's Chinese dinner!

FITTING IN YOUR FAVORITE RECIPES

Your registered dietitian can help you plan menus around a special recipe or food you want to try. Doing so requires some advice because the exchanges called for in the recipe may not be exactly those that your meal plan specifies. Say, for example, that you are using the meal plan above, which calls for 2 Starch/ Bread exchanges, 3 Lean Meat exchanges, and 1 Vegetable exchange. The main course recipe you'd like to prepare has 2 Vegetable exchanges and 2 Lean Meat exchanges. Your dietitian can give you advice on "borrowing" the carbohydrate you need from some other category. If you cut your fruit portion by one-third, for example, you could have the main course.

You'll find your menu file will build quickly if you jot down and keep your favorite combinations. In general, you'll start with the dish you're interested in making, then build around it.

Let exchanges stimulate your imagination and tempt you to experiment with new foods.

7 ◇ RECIPES

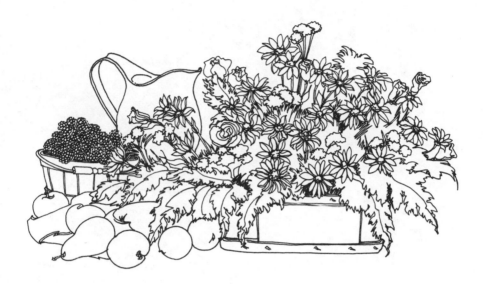

Appetizers

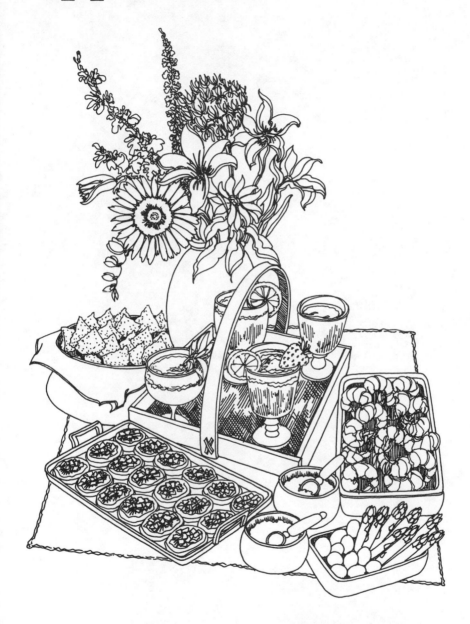

Crudités with Minted Cucumber Dip

Yield: 1½ cups (8 servings)	Nutrient Content per Serving			
Serving Size: 3 tablespoons	CAL	31	Na	22 (mg)
dip plus ½ cup raw vegetables	PRO	2 (gm)	K	238 (mg)
Exchanges:	Fat	0.5 (gm)	Fiber	2 (gm)
Vegetable 1.0	CHO	5 (gm)	Chol	2 (mg)

Ingredients

        1 8-OUNCE CARTON PLAIN LOW-FAT YOGURT
        ⅓ CUP FINELY CHOPPED CUCUMBER (WITH PEEL)
        2 TABLESPOONS GRATED ONION
        1 TABLESPOON CHOPPED FRESH MINT OR 1 TEASPOON
            DRIED MINT
        1 TEASPOON SUGAR
            HOLLOWED-OUT PEPPER, SQUASH, OR RED
            CABBAGE
            FLOWERING COLE (SALAD SAVOY)

Crudités as desired

        JICAMA STICKS
        PEELED BABY CARROTS WITH TOPS
        SUGAR SNAP PEAS
        BROCCOLI FLORETS
        YELLOW SQUASH AND ZUCCHINI STICKS OR WHOLE
        BABY SQUASH
        CHERRY TOMATOES
        FRESH MINT SPRIGS (OPTIONAL)

Method

1. Combine yogurt, cucumber, onion, mint, and sugar.
   Refrigerate until serving.
2. Place dip in hollowed-out pepper, squash, or red cabbage.
   Line a basket with flowering cole or lettuce leaves. Arrange
   crudités attractively around dip. Garnish dip with mint sprigs,
   if desired.

Black Bean and Cilantro Spread

Yield: 1¼ cups (10 servings)   Nutrient Content per Serving

Serving Size: 2 tablespoons

Exchanges:

Starch/Bread 0.5

CAL	46	Na	55 (mg)
PRO	3 (gm)	K	116 (mg)
Fat	0.6 (gm)	Fiber	2 (gm)
CHO	8 (gm)	Chol	0 (mg)

Ingredients

     1 CAN (15 OR 16 OUNCES) BLACK BEANS, RINSED AND
       DRAINED
     2 TEASPOONS LIME JUICE
     1 TEASPOON OLIVE OIL
 ¼–½ TEASPOON HOT PEPPER SAUCE
     ¼ CUP FRESH CILANTRO LEAVES
     2 TABLESPOONS FINELY DICED RED ONION

Method

1. Place beans, lime juice, oil, and pepper sauce in food processor fitted with steel blade. Process until puréed, scraping down sides once.
2. Add cilantro; process just until coarsely chopped and well mixed. Stir in red onion. Serve at room temperature as a spread for crackers or toast points.

Picante Potato Skins

Yield: 1 dozen (12 servings)
Serving Size: 1 potato skin
Exchanges:
Starch/Bread   0.5
Fat   0.5

Nutrient Content per Serving

CAL	64	Na	61 (mg)
PRO	2 (gm)	K	94 (mg)
Fat	3.1 (gm)	Fiber	0.4 (gm)
CHO	7 (gm)	Chol	7 (mg)

Ingredients

   3 BAKING POTATOES (ABOUT 1 POUND TOTAL
     WEIGHT)
   2 TABLESPOONS PREPARED SALSA OR PICANTE SAUCE
   1 TABLESPOON MARGARINE, MELTED
   ¾ CUP (3 OUNCES) SHREDDED MONTEREY JACK
     CHEESE WITH JALAPEÑOS

Method

1. Preheat oven to 400°F.
2. Wash potatoes and poke with tip of knife in several places. Bake 1 hour or until tender; cool.
3. Cut potatoes in half lengthwise. Carefully scoop out pulp, leaving ¼-inch-thick shells. (Reserve pulp for another use.)
4. Cut each shell in half lengthwise; place on foil-lined cookie sheet. Combine salsa and margarine; brush over insides of shells. Bake until crisp, about 15 minutes.
5. Sprinkle with cheese; return to oven 5 minutes or until cheese is melted. Serve warm.

Note: Potatoes should not be microwaved for this recipe as the skins become too soft.

Polenta Canapés

Yield: 1 dozen
Serving Size: 1 canapé
Exchanges:
Starch/Bread   0.5
Fat   0.5

Nutrient Content per Serving

CAL	69	*Na	96 (mg)
PRO	3 (gm)	K	45 (mg)
Fat	3.5 (gm)	Fiber	0.7 (gm)
CHO	7 (gm)	Chol	4 (mg)

*Add 44 mg if optional salt is used.

Ingredients

    1 CUP WATER
    1 CUP REDUCED-SODIUM CHICKEN BROTH
    ½ CUP YELLOW CORNMEAL
    ¼ TEASPOON SALT (OPTIONAL)
    1 TABLESPOON OLIVE OIL
    4 DRAINED MARINATED ARTICHOKE HEARTS,
       QUARTERED
    3 SLICES (3 OUNCES) PART-SKIM MOZZARELLA
       CHEESE

Method

1. Combine water, broth, cornmeal and salt, if desired, in sauce-pan. Bring to a boil, stirring constantly. Simmer 10–12 minutes over low heat, or until thickened, stirring frequently. Stir in oil.
2. Pour into 8-inch square dish or pan and chill until firm.
3. Cut into 12 squares. Place on jelly-roll pan or cookie sheet. Place ¼ artichoke heart over each square. Cut cheese into 24 thin strips. Cross 2 strips of cheese over artichoke heart, forming an X.
4. Broil 5–6 inches from heat source until cheese is melted and polenta is heated through, about 3 minutes.

Method-Microwave

1. Combine water, broth, cornmeal and salt, if desired, in

2½-quart microwave-safe casserole dish. Cook uncovered on high power 7–9 minutes, stirring each 2 minutes with wire whisk, until thickened. Stir in oil.

2. Pour into 8-inch square dish or pan; chill until firm or up to 2 days.
3. At serving time, cut into 12 squares. Place 6 squares in a ring on microwave-safe plate. Cook on high power 30 seconds to heat. Place ¼ artichoke heart over each square. Cut cheese into 24 thin strips. Cross 2 strips of cheese over artichoke heart, forming an X.
4. Cook on high power 1 minute or until cheese is melted and polenta is heated through.

Rye Breadsticks

Yield: 38 breadsticks

Serving Size: 2 breadsticks

Exchanges:

Starch/Bread 0.5

Fat 0.5

Nutrient Content per Serving

CAL	64	Na	126 (mg)
PRO	2 (gm)	K	27 (mg)
Fat	2.6 (gm)	Fiber	0.6 (gm)
CHO	9 (gm)	Chol	0 (mg)

Ingredients

1 LOAF RYE BREAD (1½ POUNDS, 12 INCHES LONG), UNSLICED

¼ CUP MARGARINE, MELTED

Method

1. Preheat oven to 350°F.
2. Cut crusts from bread. Cut lengthwise into ½-inch slices with long, serrated knife. Cut each slice lengthwise into ½-inch slices, forming sticks. Cut sticks in half crosswise, forming 6-inch breadsticks.
3. Transfer to cookie sheets. Brush lightly on all sides with margarine. Bake 15–20 minutes or until crisp.

Note: For garlic breadsticks, add 2 cloves crushed garlic to margarine when melting.

Cucumber Cups with Horseradish

Yield: 18 appetizers	Nutrient Content per Serving			
Serving Size: 2 cups	CAL	32	Na	45 (mg)
Exchanges:	PRO	1 (gm)	K	44 (mg)
Fat 0.5	Fat	2.6 (gm)	Fiber	0.4 (gm)
	CHO	1 (gm)	Chol	7 (mg)

Ingredients

2 OUNCES REDUCED-FAT CREAM CHEESE (NEUFCHÂ-
TEL), SOFTENED
2 TABLESPOONS REDUCED-CALORIE MAYONNAISE
1 TABLESPOON WELL-DRAINED PREPARED
HORSERADISH*
1 LARGE CUCUMBER (12 OUNCES), PREFERABLY
SEEDLESS (EUROPEAN), UNPEELED
SMALL PARSLEY OR DILL SPRIGS

Method

1. Combine cream cheese, mayonnaise, and horseradish; chill at least 30 minutes.
2. Score cucumber decoratively all over lengthwise with the tines of a fork. Cut crosswise into ½-inch slices. With melon baller or ½ teaspoon measuring spoon, scoop out small hollow at one end, leaving a cup but not cutting through to bottom.
3. Transfer cream cheese mixture to pastry bag fitted with fluted tip. Pipe (or spoon, if pastry bag is not available) cheese mixture into cucumber cups. Garnish with parsley sprigs.

*Beet horseradish gives these appetizers a lovely color contrast. If using regular horseradish, sprinkle lightly with paprika for added color. This is easy to prepare a few hours ahead.

Honey-Mustard Chicken Wings

Yield: 6 servings	Nutrient Content per Serving			
Serving Size: 2 chicken wings	CAL	99	Na	104 (mg)
Exchanges:	PRO	11 (gm)	K	90 (mg)
Starch/Bread 0.5	Fat	2.5 (gm)	Fiber	0.1 (gm)
Meat, lean 1.0	CHO	7 (gm)	Chol	33 (mg)

Ingredients

> 1 TABLESPOON SPICY BROWN MUSTARD OR PREPARED
> MUSTARD WITH HORSERADISH
> 1 TABLESPOON HONEY
> ⅓ CUP PLAIN DRY BREAD CRUMBS
> 12 CHICKEN WING DRUMETTES, SKINNED (1 POUND)*
> NONSTICK VEGETABLE SPRAY
> HUNGARIAN PAPRIKA, PREFERABLY HOT
> (OPTIONAL)

Method

1. Heat oven to 375°F.
2. Combine mustard and honey in small bowl. Place bread crumbs in another shallow bowl. Brush each drumette with mustard mixture; let excess drip back into bowl. Roll in bread crumbs; shake off excess.
3. Place on cookie sheet that has been sprayed with vegetable spray. Sprinkle with paprika, if desired. Bake 30 minutes or until crisp. Serve warm or at room temperature.

Method-Microwave

1. Prepare drumettes as directed above. Place in spoke fashion with meaty portions toward outer edge of plate.
2. Cover with paper towel. Cook on high power 4 minutes. Turn over; continue to cook 4–5 minutes or until crisp. Let stand uncovered 3 minutes. Serve warm or at room temperature.

Note: Drumettes are the meaty drumstick portion of the chicken wing often packaged separately. If not available, purchase whole chicken wings, cut off drumettes, and reserve remaining wing sections for Homemade Chicken Broth (page 118) or another use.

* Recipe may be easily doubled to serve 12. If using microwave method, cook only 12 drumettes at one time as directed above.

Curried Turkey and Asparagus Rolls

Yield: 12 servings
Serving Size: 1 roll
Exchanges:
Meat, lean   1.0
Vegetable   1.0

Nutrient Content per Serving

CAL	88	Na	128 (mg)
PRO	11 (gm)	K	159 (mg)
Fat	3.6 (gm)	Fiber	0.3 (gm)
CHO	4 (gm)	Chol	34 (mg)

Ingredients

1 TUB (8 OUNCES) REDUCED-FAT CREAM CHEESE (NEUFCHÁTEL)
2 TABLESPOONS CHOPPED MANGO CHUTNEY
1 TEASPOON CURRY POWDER
12 SLICES LEAN TURKEY BREAST (12 OUNCES)
12 4-INCH ASPARAGUS SPEARS, COOKED CRISP-TENDER

Method

1. Combine cream cheese, chutney, and curry powder. Spread evenly over turkey slices. Starting just below tip of asparagus, roll prepared turkey slice around length of asparagus spear in a spiral fashion.

Variation: Twenty-four ripe pear or apple slices may be substituted for the asparagus; cut turkey strips in half before rolling.

Santa Fe Seviche

Yield: 6 servings
Serving Size: ⅙ recipe
Exchanges:
Meat, lean 2.0
Fat 0.5

Nutrient Content per Serving

CAL	129	Na	42 (mg)
PRO	14 (gm)	K	387 (mg)
Fat	7.4 (gm)	Fiber	0.5 (gm)
CHO	2 (gm)	Chol	32 (mg)

Ingredients

- 1 POUND PERCH OR COD FILLETS, CUT INTO ½-INCH CHUNKS
- ½ CUP PLUS 2 TABLESPOONS FRESH LIME JUICE
- 3 TABLESPOONS OLIVE OIL
- 1 CLOVE GARLIC, MINCED
- 3 TABLESPOONS SLICED GREEN ONIONS WITH TOPS
- 1 TABLESPOON CHOPPED FRESH HOT PEPPER SUCH AS ANAHEIM OR JALAPEÑO
- 2 TABLESPOONS CHOPPED ROASTED RED PEPPER OR PIMIENTO
- 3 TABLESPOONS CHOPPED FRESH CILANTRO
- 6 LARGE BOSTON OR RED LEAF LETTUCE LEAVES

Method

1. Place fish chunks in glass bowl so they fit in one layer. Pour ½ cup lime juice over all. Push down so fish is covered with juice. Cover and refrigerate 6 hours or overnight, until fish is opaque.
2. Pour off lime juice. Combine remaining 2 tablespoons lime juice, oil, and garlic. Toss fish with oil mixture and remaining ingredients except lettuce leaves. Serve immediately or chill up to 1 hour before serving. Serve on lettuce leaves.

Note: Fish will "cook" and become firm in lime marinade. This is a great "make ahead" dish for the cocktail buffet table. Fresh, very fresh, fish is essential.

Greek-Style Marinated Mushrooms

Yield: 3⅓ cups (10 servings)   Nutrient Content per Serving

Serving Size: ⅓ cup

		CAL	37	Na	1 (mg)

Exchanges:

		PRO	1 (gm)	K	164 (mg)
Vegetable	1.0	Fat	2.9 (gm)	Fiber	1.8 (gm)
Fat	0.5	CHO	3 (gm)	Chol	0 (mg)

Ingredients

   3 CLOVES GARLIC, MINCED
   ⅓ CUP EXTRA VIRGIN OLIVE OIL
   ¼ CUP RED WINE VINEGAR
   1 TABLESPOON WHOLE CORIANDER SEEDS
   ½ TEASPOON DRIED THYME LEAVES
   ½ TEASPOON DRIED OREGANO LEAVES
   ¼ TEASPOON FRESHLY GROUND BLACK PEPPER
   1½ POUNDS SMALL TO MEDIUM MUSHROOMS, STEMS
      TRIMMED FLAT

Method

1. Sauté garlic in oil in 10-inch sauté pan 2 minutes. Add remaining ingredients except mushrooms; bring to a boil.
2. Add mushrooms; cover and simmer over low heat 5 minutes or until mushrooms are tender, stirring occasionally.
3. Cover and refrigerate 1–7 days before serving. Drain off and discard marinade before serving.

Method-Microwave

1. Combine oil and garlic in 2-quart microwave-safe casserole. Cover and cook on high power 2 minutes. Add remaining ingredients except mushrooms. Cover and cook on high power 2 minutes.
2. Add mushrooms; toss to coat well. Cover and cook on high power 5 minutes, stirring twice. Proceed as directed in step 3 above.

Baby Corn in Jalapeño Vinaigrette

Yield: 8 servings
Serving Size: ⅛ recipe
Exchanges:
Starch/Bread   0.5
Fat   0.5

Nutrient Content per Serving

CAL	58	Na	93 (mg)
PRO	1 (gm)	K	74 (mg)
Fat	3.5 (gm)	Fiber	2.0 (gm)
CHO	7 (gm)	Chol	0 (mg)

Ingredients

1 16-OUNCE CAN OR 2 7-OUNCE JARS WHOLE BABY
   CORN COBS, RINSED AND DRAINED
¼ CUP CHOPPED CILANTRO
¼ CUP RED OR WHITE WINE VINEGAR
2 TABLESPOONS OLIVE OIL
1 SMALL JALAPEÑO PEPPER, MINCED

Method

1. Combine all ingredients in glass dish; marinate covered and refrigerate at least 2 hours or overnight. Drain before serving. Serve chilled or at room temperature. May be refrigerated up to 3 days.

Note: Baby corn is grown in Thailand. During the peak growing season, some specialty produce growers offer it fresh. If you are lucky enough to find it, substitute 8 ounces fresh for canned.

Tex-Mex Bean Dip

Yield: 1¼–1½ cups
Serving Size: 2 tablespoons
dip plus 3 chips
Exchanges:
Starch/Bread   1.0
Fat   0.5

Nutrient Content per Serving

CAL	108	Na	162 (mg)
PRO	4 (gm)	K	230 (mg)
Fat	3.5 (gm)	Fiber	3.6 (gm)
CHO	16 (gm)	Chol	0 (mg)

Ingredients

1 CLOVE GARLIC, MINCED
1 TABLESPOON OLIVE OIL
1 16-OUNCE CAN PINTO BEANS, RINSED AND DRAINED
⅓ CUP PREPARED SALSA OR PICANTE SAUCE
1 TEASPOON CHILI POWDER
1 TEASPOON GROUND CUMIN
¼ CUP THINLY SLICED GREEN ONIONS
¼ CUP CHOPPED CILANTRO
24–30 TORTILLA CHIPS

Method

1. Sauté garlic in oil in medium saucepan. Add beans; coarsely mash with wooden spoon. Add salsa, chili powder, and cumin; heat through.
2. Stir in green onions and cilantro; transfer to chafing dish to keep warm for dipping. Serve with chips.

Method-Microwave

1. Combine oil and garlic in 1½-quart microwave-safe casserole. Cover and cook on high power 1 minute. Add beans; coarsely mash with wooden spoon. Add salsa, chili powder, and cumin; cover and cook on high power until hot, stirring once, about 4 minutes. Proceed as directed in step 2 above.

Note: To lower sodium in this recipe even further, look for low-salt or unsalted tortilla chips in your market.

Soups

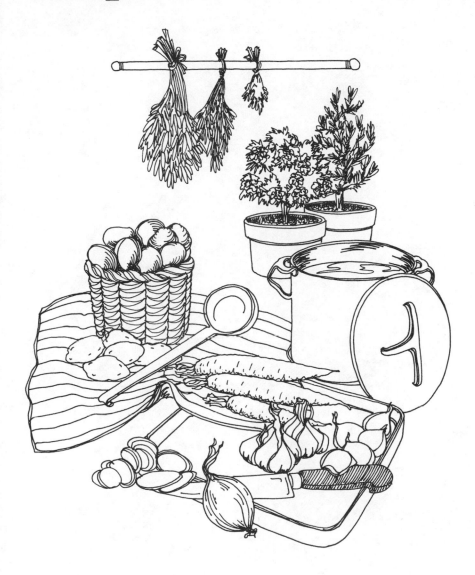

Summer Garden Soup

Yield: 6 cups (6 servings)	Nutrient Content per Serving
Serving Size: 1 cup	CAL 64 Na 48 (mg)
Exchanges:	PRO 4 (gm) K 570 (mg)
Vegetable 2.0	Fat 0.7 (gm) Fiber 1 (gm)
	CHO 12 (gm) Chol 2 (mg)

Ingredients

> 4 CUPS NO-SALT-ADDED TOMATO JUICE
> 1 8-OUNCE CARTON PLAIN LOW-FAT YOGURT
> 2 TABLESPOONS GRATED ONION OR CHOPPED CHIVES
> ½ TEASPOON HOT PEPPER SAUCE
> 2 RIPE TOMATOES, SEEDED AND FINELY DICED (8 OUNCES, 1½ CUPS)
> 1 SMALL CUCUMBER, SEEDED AND FINELY DICED (4 OUNCES, 1 CUP)
> 2 TABLESPOONS FINELY CHOPPED FRESH BASIL OR 2 TEASPOONS DRIED BASIL
> 2 TABLESPOONS CHOPPED PARSLEY

Method

1. Whisk together tomato juice, yogurt, onion, and pepper sauce.
2. Stir in tomatoes, cucumber, and basil. Chill at least 2 hours or overnight.
3. Ladle into chilled soup bowls; sprinkle with parsley.

Note: Now there is no excuse for letting the vegetables in the garden go unpicked. This soup will keep several days in the refrigerator and travels well to picnics.

Creole-Style Vegetable Soup

Yield: 5 cups (5 servings)	Nutrient Content per Serving			
Serving Size: 1 cup	CAL	72	Na	72 (mg)
Exchanges:	PRO	3 (gm)	K	328 (mg)
Vegetable 2.0	Fat	1.8 (gm)	Fiber	2 (gm)
Fat 0.5	CHO	13 (gm)	Chol	0 (mg)

Ingredients

> 1 LARGE ONION, COARSELY CHOPPED (8 OUNCES)
> ½ CUP SLICED CELERY (2 OUNCES)
> 1 CLOVE GARLIC, MINCED
> 1 TEASPOON OLIVE OIL
> 2 CUPS REDUCED-SODIUM CHICKEN BROTH
> 1 14½-OUNCE CAN NO-SALT-ADDED TOMATOES, UN-DRAINED AND COARSELY CHOPPED
> 1 CUP SLICED CARROTS (4 OUNCES)
> 1 TEASPOON THYME
> ½ TEASPOON HOT PEPPER SAUCE
> ¼ TEASPOON FRESHLY GROUND BLACK PEPPER
> 1 CUP CHOPPED CABBAGE (3 OUNCES)
> 1 SMALL GREEN BELL PEPPER, CHOPPED (4 OUNCES)
> 1 TABLESPOON LEMON JUICE

Method

1. Sauté onion, celery, and garlic in oil in large saucepan.
2. Stir in broth, tomatoes, carrots, thyme, pepper sauce, and pepper. Bring to a boil; reduce heat. Cover and simmer 25 minutes.
3. Add cabbage and bell pepper; cover and continue to simmer 10 minutes or until vegetables are tender. Stir in lemon juice.

Method-Microwave

1. Toss onion, celery, and garlic with oil in 2½-quart microwave-safe casserole dish. Cover and cook on high power 3 minutes.
2. Stir in broth, tomatoes, carrots, thyme, pepper sauce, and

pepper. Cover and cook on high power until boiling, 6–7 minutes. Reduce heat to medium power and cook 18–20 minutes.
3. Stir in cabbage and bell pepper; cover and continue to cook 8–10 minutes or until vegetables are tender. Stir in lemon juice.

Note: Soups keep up to a week refrigerated. Make on a relaxed weekend and store for quick meals during the week. Microwave in soup bowls for easy cleanup.

Chilled Curried Tomato Soup

Yield: 3 cups (4 servings)
Serving Size: ¾ cup
Exchanges:
Starch/Bread   1.0

Nutrient Content per Serving

CAL	85	Na	273 (mg)
PRO	5 (gm)	K	382 (mg)
Fat	1.7 (gm)	Fiber	1 (gm)
CHO	14 (gm)	Chol	3 (mg)

Ingredients

1 28-OUNCE CAN PLUM TOMATOES, DRAINED AND COARSELY CHOPPED
1 10½-OUNCE CAN REDUCED-SODIUM CHICKEN BROTH OR 1⅓ CUPS HOMEMADE (PAGE 118)
1 TABLESPOON BROWN SUGAR
2 TEASPOONS CURRY POWDER
1 8-OUNCE CARTON PLAIN LOW-FAT YOGURT
2 TABLESPOONS CHOPPED FRESH MINT LEAVES (OPTIONAL)

Method

1. Combine tomatoes, broth, sugar, and curry powder in saucepan. Simmer uncovered 10 minutes; cool to room temperature.
2. Purée in food processor fitted with steel blade. Strain. Transfer to large bowl. Whisk in yogurt. Chill until cold. Sprinkle with mint leaves before serving, if desired.

Tangy Butternut Soup

	Nutrient Content per Serving		
Yield: 7 cups (7 servings)			
Serving Size: 1 cup	CAL 82	Na	104 (mg)
Exchanges:	PRO 4 (gm)	K	282 (mg)
Starch/Bread 1.0	Fat 2.7 (gm)	Fiber	2.8 (gm)
	CHO 12 (gm)	Chol	2 (mg)

Ingredients

1 TABLESPOON MARGARINE
1½ CUPS CHOPPED ONION
1¾ POUNDS BUTTERNUT OR ACORN SQUASH, PEELED,
    SEEDED, AND CUT INTO 1-INCH PIECES (4 CUPS)
2 CUPS REDUCED-SODIUM CHICKEN BROTH
1 CUP WATER
¼ TEASPOON FRESHLY GRATED NUTMEG
1¾ CUPS LOW-FAT BUTTERMILK
    FRESHLY GRATED NUTMEG

Method

1. Melt margarine in large saucepan over medium heat. Sauté onion in margarine until tender, about 5 minutes.
2. Add squash, broth, and water. Cover and simmer until squash is very tender, about 25 minutes.
3. Transfer in batches to food professor fitted with steel blade and purée until smooth. Stir in nutmeg. Chill until cold.
4. Just before serving, stir in buttermilk; garnish with freshly grated nutmeg.

Method-Microwave

1. Place margarine in 3-quart microwave-safe casserole dish. Cook on high power until melted, about 45 seconds. Add onion; toss to coat with margarine.
2. Cover and cook on high power 3 minutes. Stir in squash, broth, and water. Cover and cook until squash is very tender, about 22–24 minutes. Proceed as in steps 3 and 4 above.

Lentil Soup with Ham

Yield: 7 cups (7 servings)
Serving Size: 1 cup
Exchanges:
Starch/Bread   1.0

Nutrient Content per Serving

CAL	83	Na	17 (mg)
PRO	7 (gm)	K	231 (mg)
Fat	1.6 (gm)	Fiber	3 (gm)
CHO	11 (gm)	Chol	8 (mg)

Ingredients

    1 CUP BROWN LENTILS (8 OUNCES)
    6 CUPS WATER
    1 SMALL SMOKED HAM HOCK (8 OUNCES)
    1 LARGE ONION, CHOPPED (8 OUNCES, 2 CUPS)
    2 CLOVES GARLIC, MINCED
    1 TEASPOON DRIED THYME LEAVES
    1 BAY LEAF
    ½ TEASPOON FRESHLY GROUND BLACK PEPPER

Method

1. Place lentils in large saucepan or Dutch oven. Add remaining ingredients.
2. Bring to a boil; reduce heat. Cover and simmer until lentils are tender, about 45 minutes, stirring occasionally.
3. Remove ham hock. Chop meat, discarding fat and bone. If thicker soup is desired, purée half of lentil mixture in food processor fitted with steel blade, discarding bay leaf.
4. Return ham to soup; heat through.

Method-Microwave

1. Place lentils in 3-quart microwave-safe casserole dish. Add remaining ingredients.
2. Cover and cook on high power until boiling, 12–14 minutes. Reduce power to medium and continue to cook until lentils are tender, 40–45 minutes, stirring twice.
3. Proceed as directed in step 3 above.
4. Heat soup on high power 1–2 minutes.

Wisconsin Onion-Beer Soup

Yield: 7 cups (7 servings)
Serving Size: 1 cup
Exchanges:

		Nutrient Content per Serving			
		CAL	168	Na	241 (mg)
		PRO	7 (gm)	K	92 (mg)
Starch/Bread	1.0	Fat	7.0 (gm)	Fiber	2.5 (gm)
Vegetable	1.0	CHO	19 (gm)	Chol	8 (mg)
Fat	1.5				

Ingredients

    2 TABLESPOONS MARGARINE
    1 POUND YELLOW ONIONS, THINLY SLICED (4 CUPS)
    3 TABLESPOONS FLOUR
    ¼ TEASPOON FRESHLY GRATED NUTMEG
    4 CUPS REDUCED-SODIUM BEEF BROTH
    1 12-OUNCE BOTTLE OR CAN BEER
    7 ½-INCH SLICES FRENCH BREAD (2-INCH DIAMETER)
    1 TEASPOON OLIVE OIL
    ¾ CUP (3 OUNCES) SHREDDED REDUCED-FAT SHARP
      CHEDDAR CHEESE

Method

1. Melt margarine in large saucepan. Sauté onions over medium-low heat until golden and very tender, about 15–20 minutes, stirring frequently.
2. Sprinkle with flour and nutmeg; cook 1 minute.
3. Stir in broth and beer; bring to a boil. Reduce heat; simmer uncovered 25 minutes, stirring occasionally.
4. While soup is simmering, brush bread lightly with oil. Broil or toast until crisp. Ladle soup into bowls; top each with one crouton. Sprinkle with cheese.

Method-Microwave

1. Place margarine in 3-quart microwave-safe casserole dish. Cook on high power until melted, about 1 minute. Toss onions in

margarine. Cover and cook on high power 5 minutes. Reduce power to medium and cook 15 minutes, stirring once.
2. Stir in flour and nutmeg; cook on high power 1 minute.
3. Stir in broth and beer; cover and cook on high power until boiling, about 5 minutes. Stir. Reduce power to medium and cook 20 minutes).

Creamy Carrot Soup

Yield: 6 cups (6 servings)	Nutrient Content per Serving			
Serving Size: 1 cup	CAL	117	Na	161 (mg)
Exchanges:	PRO	5 (gm)	K	334 (mg)
Starch/Bread 1.0	Fat	3.4 (gm)	Fiber	3 (gm)
Fat 0.5	CHO	17 (gm)	Chol	3 (mg)

Ingredients

¾ POUND THINLY SLICED CARROTS (ABOUT 2 CUPS)
1 SMALL ONION, CHOPPED (4 OUNCES)
1 TABLESPOON MARGARINE
2 CUPS REDUCED-SODIUM CHICKEN BROTH
1 LARGE RED BELL PEPPER, CHOPPED (7 OUNCES, 1¼ CUPS)
1 MEDIUM POTATO, PEELED AND CHOPPED (8 OUNCES, ABOUT 1 CUP)
½ TEASPOON HOT PEPPER SAUCE
2 CUPS LOW-FAT BUTTERMILK
2 TABLESPOONS CHOPPED CHIVES

Method

1. Sauté carrots and onion in margarine in large saucepan over medium heat 8 minutes.
2. Add broth, red pepper, potato, and pepper sauce. Bring to a boil; reduce heat. Cover; simmer 25 minutes or until vegetables are tender.

(continued on page 114)

3. Transfer to food processor in batches. Process until very smooth (mixture will be somewhat thick.) Chill at least 4 hours or overnight.
4. Stir in buttermilk just before serving; garnish with chives.

Method-Microwave

1. Cook margarine in 2-quart microwave-safe casserole on high power until melted, about 45 seconds. Toss carrots and onion with margarine. Cover; cook on high power 3–4 minutes.
2. Stir in broth, red pepper, potato, and pepper sauce. Cover; cook on high power until boiling, about 6 minutes. Reduce power to medium and continue cooking 20–22 minutes or until vegetables are tender, stirring once.
3. Proceed as directed above in steps 3 and 4.

Note: This soup may be made ahead and frozen up to 3 months. Freeze before adding buttermilk. Thaw in refrigerator overnight; stir well and add buttermilk just before serving.

Chicken Soup with Lime and Cilantro

Yield: 6 servings (4½ cups)   Nutrient Content per Serving

Serving Size: ¾ cup

CAL	67	Na	53 (mg)
PRO	10 (gm)	K	–11 (mg)
Fat	1.9 (gm)	Fiber	0 (gm)
CHO	2 (gm)	Chol	23 (mg)

Exchanges:

Meat, lean   1.0

Ingredients

   4 CUPS REDUCED-SODIUM CHICKEN BROTH
   1 WHOLE CHICKEN BREAST, SKINNED, BONED, AND
     SPLIT
   3 TABLESPOONS FRESH LIME JUICE
   ¼ CUP COARSELY CHOPPED CILANTRO LEAVES

Method

1. Bring broth to a simmer in large saucepan. Add chicken; cover and simmer over low heat until chicken is just cooked through, about 8–10 minutes.
2. Remove and shred chicken. Return to broth with lime juice. Ladle into soup bowls; sprinkle with cilantro.

Method-Microwave

1. Place broth in 2-quart microwave-safe casserole dish. Cover and cook on high power until boiling, about 8 minutes. Add chicken; reduce power to medium and continue to cook 8–10 minutes or until chicken is just cooked through.
2. Remove and shred chicken. Return to broth with lime juice. Ladle into soup bowls; sprinkle with cilantro.

Note: This sophisticated soup with few ingredients takes only minutes to prepare.

Tuscan Vegetable Soup with Orzo

Yield: 7 cups (7 servings)	Nutrient Content per Serving			
Serving size: 1 cup	CAL	100	*Na	698 (mg)
Exchanges:	PRO	4 (gm)	K	225 (mg)
Starch/Bread 1.0	Fat	2.9 (gm)	Fiber	2.7 (gm)
Fat 0.5	CHO	15 (gm)	Chol	2 (mg)

*Add 76 mg if optional salt is used.

Ingredients

  1 LARGE ONION, COARSELY CHOPPED (6 OUNCES)

  2 CLOVES GARLIC, MINCED

  2 TEASPOONS OLIVE OIL

  8 OUNCES MUSHROOMS, SLICED

  1 CUP DRY WHITE WINE

  1 12½-OUNCE CAN REDUCED-SODIUM CHICKEN BROTH

  2 CUPS WATER

  ¼ TEASPOON SALT (OPTIONAL)

  ¼ TEASPOON FRESHLY GROUND BLACK PEPPER

  1 LARGE ZUCCHINI AND 1 LARGE YELLOW SQUASH, SLICED ½ INCH THICK, EACH SLICE QUARTERED (8 OUNCES EACH, 3 CUPS)

  ½ CUP UNCOOKED ORZO (RICE-SHAPED PASTA) (3 OUNCES)

  ¼ CUP CHOPPED FRESH BASIL, MARJORAM, OREGANO, OR ITALIAN PARSLEY LEAVES OR 1 TEASPOON EACH DRIED BASIL AND MARJORAM, CRUSHED

  ¼ CUP FRESHLY GRATED PARMESAN CHEESE (1 OUNCE)

Method

1. Sauté onion and garlic in oil in large saucepan or Dutch oven over medium heat until tender, about 4 minutes. Add mushrooms; sauté 2 minutes.
2. Add wine, broth, and water; bring to a boil. Reduce heat; cover and simmer 10 minutes.

3. Add squash and orzo; cover and continue to simmer until pasta and squash are tender, about 10–15 minutes.
4. Remove from heat; stir in basil. Sprinkle with cheese.

Method-Microwave

1. Toss onion and garlic with oil in 2½-quart microwave-safe casserole dish. Cover and cook on high power 3–4 minutes. Stir in mushrooms; cook, covered, 2 minutes more.
2. Add wine, broth, and water. Cover and cook on high power until boiling, about 5–6 minutes. Stir; reduce power to medium and cook 6 minutes.
3. Stir in squash and orzo; cover and continue to cook on medium power until pasta and squash are tender, about 15–18 minutes.
4. Remove from heat; stir in basil. Sprinkle with cheese.

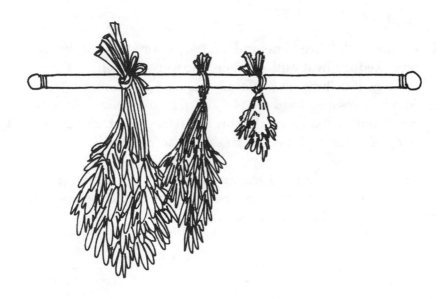

Homemade Chicken Broth

Yield: 5 cups (10 servings)
Serving Size: ½ cup

Nutrient Content per Serving

CAL	16	Na	28 (mg)
PRO	1 (gm)	K	86 (mg)
Fat	0.8 (gm)	Fiber	0 (gm)
CHO	1 (gm)	Chol	1 (mg)

Ingredients

2 QUARTS WATER
3 POUNDS CHICKEN BACKS, NECKS, AND/OR WINGS
3 CUPS COARSELY CHOPPED ONION (12 OUNCES)
2 CUPS COARSELY CHOPPED CARROTS (8 OUNCES, 4 MEDIUM)
8 WHOLE PEPPERCORNS
½ CUP PARSLEY SPRIGS
2 BAY LEAVES

Method

1. Combine all ingredients in Dutch oven or stockpot. Bring to a boil. Reduce heat and simmer uncovered 2 hours, skimming foam as it collects on surface.
2. Strain, pressing hard on solids. Discard solids. Refrigerate broth until fat is congealed on top. Discard fat. Store covered and refrigerated 3 days or freeze up to 6 months.

Note: Buying whole chickens and cutting them up is very economical, especially when the backs, necks, and wings can be frozen and saved for this versatile broth.

Vegetable Broth

Yield: 4½ cups (9 servings)
Serving Size: ½ cup

Nutrient Content per Serving			
CAL	2	Na	2 (mg)
PRO	0 (gm)	K	24 (mg)
Fat	0 (gm)	Fiber	0 (gm)
CHO	1 (gm)	Chol	0 (mg)

Ingredients

> 1 QUART WATER
> 2 LARGE CARROTS, COARSELY CHOPPED (8 OUNCES)
> 1 LARGE ONION, COARSELY CHOPPED (10 OUNCES)
> 2 LARGE RIBS CELERY WITH LEAVES, COARSELY
>   CHOPPED (6 OUNCES)
> 1 MEDIUM TOMATO, CHOPPED (6 OUNCES)
> ½ CUP PARSLEY SPRIGS
> 1 BAY LEAF

Method

1. Combine all ingredients in saucepan. Cover and heat to a boil, then reduce heat and simmer 20 minutes. Strain, pressing on solids. Use in place of chicken broth in soups, ragouts, stews, and sauces or as a flavorful broth for quickly cooked vegetables.

Method-Microwave

1. Combine all ingredients in 2½-quart microwave-safe casserole dish. Cover with lid or vented plastic wrap.
2. Cook on high power 10 minutes. Reduce power to medium and continue cooking 20 minutes. Strain, pressing on solids.

Note: Broth may be frozen in small quantities to use as needed in sauces, soups, and stews.

Oriental Chicken Soup in Cantaloupe

Yield: 2 servings
Serving Size: ½ recipe
Exchanges:
Meat, lean   1.5
Fruit   1.0

Nutrient Content per Serving

CAL	140	Na	369 (mg)
PRO	10 (gm)	K	488 (mg)
Fat	4.2 (gm)	Fiber	1.7 (gm)
CHO	17 (gm)	Chol	19 (mg)

Ingredients

1 LARGE DRIED SHIITAKE MUSHROOM
1 10½-OUNCE CAN REDUCED-SODIUM CHICKEN BROTH OR 1⅓ CUPS HOMEMADE (PAGE 118)
⅓ CUP SHREDDED COOKED CHICKEN OR TURKEY
1 TABLESPOON REDUCED-SODIUM SOY SAUCE
1 TEASPOON FINELY SHREDDED FRESH GINGERROOT
½ TEASPOON ORIENTAL SESAME OIL
1 LARGE RIPE CANTALOUPE (2½ POUNDS), AT ROOM TEMPERATURE
1 TABLESPOON CHOPPED CILANTRO (OPTIONAL)

Method

1. Soak mushroom in very hot tap water to cover, about 15 minutes. Drain and discard liquid. Discard stem and slice cap thinly.
2. Combine chicken broth, sliced mushroom, chicken, soy sauce, ginger, and sesame oil in saucepan. Cover and simmer 10 minutes.
3. Cut cantaloupe in half crosswise; scoop out and discard seeds. Scoop out flesh, leaving a 1-inch border. (Reserve flesh for another use.) Set each cantaloupe half in serving bowl small enough to hold cantaloupe upright. Bring soup to a rolling boil; pour into cantaloupe halves. Let stand 5 minutes to soften cantaloupe flesh. Eat soup, scooping some cantaloupe flesh with each bite.

Method-Microwave

1. Prepare mushroom as directed in step 1 above.
2. Combine broth, sliced mushroom, chicken, soy sauce, ginger, and sesame oil in 1-quart microwave-safe bowl or measure. Cover and cook on high power 4 minutes. Reduce power to medium and continue to cook 5–6 minutes.
3. Prepare cantaloupe as directed in step 3 above. If desired, instead of letting soup stand 5 minutes to soften cantaloupe, use microwave-safe bowls and return soup in bowls to microwave oven. Cook on high power 1–2 minutes.

Corn and Red Pepper Chowder

Yield: 4 cups (4 servings)
Serving Size: 1 cup
Exchanges:
Starch/Bread   2.0

Nutrient Content per Serving

CAL	167	Na	82 (mg)
PRO	8 (gm)	K	315 (mg)
Fat	2.3 (gm)	Fiber	6.6 (gm)
CHO	32 (gm)	Chol	0 (mg)

Ingredients

1 LARGE ONION, CHOPPED
1 TABLESPOON MARGARINE
3 TABLESPOONS FLOUR
2 CUPS REDUCED-SODIUM CHICKEN BROTH OR HOMEMADE (PAGE 118)
2 CUPS FRESH OR FROZEN-AND-THAWED CORN KERNELS
1 LARGE RED BELL PEPPER, DICED
⅛ TEASPOON CAYENNE PEPPER
1 CUP SKIM MILK

(continued on page 122)

Method

1. Cook onion in margarine in large saucepan 4 minutes. Sprinkle with flour; cook and stir 1 minute. Add broth, corn, bell pepper, and cayenne. Bring to a boil; reduce heat and simmer uncovered 10 minutes, stirring occasionally. Stir in milk and heat through.

Method-Microwave

1. Place margarine in 2-quart microwave-safe casserole dish. Cook on high power until melted, 45 seconds. Toss onion with margarine; cover and cook on high power 3 minutes. Stir in flour. Stir in broth, corn, bell pepper, and cayenne. Cover and cook on high power 8 minutes. Reduce power to medium and cook 6–8 minutes, stirring once. Stir in milk.

Hot and Sour Soup

Yield: 4 servings	Nutrient Content per Serving			
Serving Size: ¼ recipe	CAL	108	Na	347 (mg)
Exchanges:	PRO	6 (gm)	K	26 (mg)
Starch/Bread 1.0	Fat	5.4 (gm)	Fiber	0.4 (gm)
Fat 1.0	CHO	10 (gm)	Chol	1 (mg)

Ingredients

    4 DRIED SHIITAKE MUSHROOMS, STEMS REMOVED
        AND DISCARDED
    1 CUP BOILING WATER
    3 CUPS REDUCED-SODIUM CHICKEN BROTH OR
        HOMEMADE (PAGE 118)
    2 TABLESPOONS REDUCED-SODIUM SOY SAUCE
    1 CUP JULIENNED OR DICED FIRM BEAN CURD (TOFU)
    ½ CUP SLIVERED CANNED BAMBOO SHOOTS, RINSED
        AND DRAINED
    3 TABLESPOONS RICE WINE VINEGAR

½ TEASPOON RED PEPPER FLAKES
2 TABLESPOONS CORNSTARCH COMBINED WITH 2
  TABLESPOONS COLD WATER
2 TEASPOONS ORIENTAL SESAME OIL
1 GREEN ONION, FINELY CHOPPED

Method

1. Soak mushrooms in boiling water 30 minutes. Strain and reserve liquid; thinly slice mushrooms.
2. Combine mushroom liquid, mushrooms, broth, and soy sauce in medium saucepan. Bring to a boil. Add bean curd, bamboo shoots, vinegar, and pepper flakes; reduce heat and simmer 5 minutes.
3. Stir in cornstarch mixture; cook and stir until thickened, about 2 minutes. Remove from heat and stir in oil. Garnish with onion.

Method-Microwave

1. Prepare mushrooms as in step 1 above.
2. Combine mushroom liquid, mushrooms, broth, and soy sauce in 2½-quart microwave-safe casserole. Cover and cook on high power until simmering, 6–8 minutes. Add bean curd, bamboo shoots, vinegar, and pepper flakes. Cover and cook on high power 5 minutes.
3. Stir in cornstarch mixture; cover and cook on high power until thickened, about 4 minutes, stirring once. Stir in oil; garnish with onion.

Note: Oriental sesame oil, found in the Oriental section of most large supermarkets, adds a great deal of flavor when stirred in after cooking. Use it to give an exotic flavor to rice or pasta side dishes.

Mushroom Barley Soup

Yield: 3 cups

Serving Size: 1 cup

Exchanges:

		Nutrient Content per Serving			
		CAL	194	*Na	164 (mg)
		PRO	8 (gm)	K	351 (mg)
Starch/Bread	1.5	Fat	6.9 (gm)	Fiber	3.5 (gm)
Fat	1.5	CHO	25 (gm)	Chol	2 (mg)

*Add 277 mg if optional salt is used.

Ingredients

1 SMALL ONION, CHOPPED
2 TABLESPOONS MARGARINE
1½ CUPS SLICED MUSHROOMS
2 TABLESPOONS ALL-PURPOSE FLOUR
1½ CUPS REDUCED-SODIUM CHICKEN BROTH OR
    HOMEMADE (PAGE 118)
1 CUP EVAPORATED SKIM MILK
¼ CUP QUICK-COOKING PEARLED BARLEY
½ TEASPOON SALT (OPTIONAL)
¼ TEASPOON FRESHLY GROUND BLACK PEPPER
1 TABLESPOON DRY SHERRY
2 TABLESPOONS CHOPPED FRESH PARSLEY

Method

1. Sauté onion in margarine until softened. Add mushrooms; sauté until tender, about 5 minutes.
2. Sprinkle with flour; cook 1 minute. Add broth, milk, barley, salt (if desired), and pepper. Cover and simmer until barley is tender, about 12 minutes, stirring occasionally. Stir in sherry; garnish with parsley.

Method-Microwave

1. Place margarine in 2½-quart microwave-safe casserole; cook on high power until melted, about 45 seconds. Toss onion

and mushrooms with margarine. Cover and cook on high power 4 minutes, stirring once.

2. Stir in flour, mixing well. Add broth, milk, barley, salt (if desired), and pepper. Cover and cook on high power until simmering, about 5 minutes. Reduce power to medium and cook until barley is tender, about 12–15 minutes, stirring once. Stir in sherry; garnish with parsley.

Salads
and Dressings

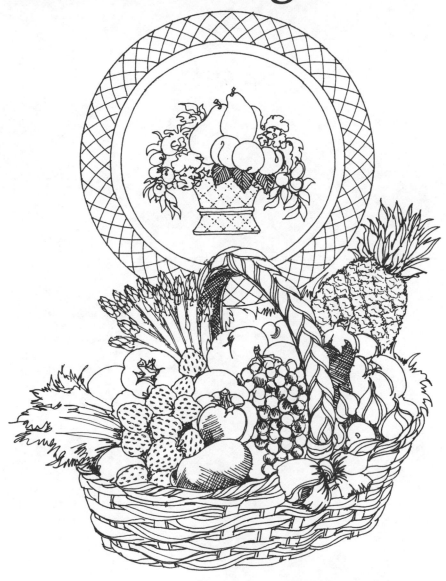

Balsamic Vinaigrette

Yield: ½ cup (8 servings)
Serving Size: 1 tablespoon
Exchanges:
Fat   1.5

Nutrient Content per Serving

CAL	61	*Na	0 (mg)
PRO	0 (gm)	K	9 (mg)
Fat	6.8 (gm)	Fiber	0 (gm)
CHO	1 (gm)	Chol	0 (mg)

*Add 33 mg if optional salt is used.

Ingredients

¼ CUP BALSAMIC VINEGAR
1 CLOVE GARLIC, MINCED
¼ TEASPOON SALT (OPTIONAL)
¼ TEASPOON FRESHLY GROUND BLACK PEPPER
¼ CUP EXTRA-VIRGIN OLIVE OIL

Method

1. Combine vinegar, garlic, salt (if desired), and pepper.
2. Whisk in oil. Will keep refrigerated 2 weeks.

Note: Best-quality olive oils are expensive, but the flavor is best appreciated in simply dressed salads. Use a less expensive olive oil for sautéing vegetables and meats.

Fresh Spinach Salad

Yield: 2 servings	Nutrient Content per Serving		
Serving Size: ½ recipe	CAL 86	*Na	35 (mg)
Exchanges:	PRO 2 (gm)	K	404 (mg)
Vegetable 1.0	Fat 7.1 (gm)	Fiber	2 (gm)
Fat 1.5	CHO 5 (gm)	Chol	0 (mg)

*Add 33 mg if optional salt is used in the Balsamic Vinaigrette.

Ingredients

> 3 CUPS PACKED TORN SPINACH LEAVES (3 OUNCES)
> 1 CUP THINLY SLICED MUSHROOMS (2 OUNCES)
> ¼ CUP THINLY SLICED RED ONION RINGS
> 2 TABLESPOONS BALSAMIC VINAIGRETTE (PAGE 129)
> FRESHLY GROUND BLACK PEPPER

Method

1. Combine spinach, mushrooms, and onion; toss with vinaigrette.
2. Serve on chilled salad plates with pepper to taste.

Curried Chicken Salad

Yield: 2 cups (4 servings)
Serving Size: ½ cup
Exchanges:

Meat, lean	2.0
Fruit	1.0

Nutrient Content per Serving

CAL	168	Na	96 (mg)
PRO	18 (gm)	K	249 (mg)
Fat	4.9 (gm)	Fiber	1 (gm)
CHO	13 (gm)	Chol	50 (mg)

Ingredients

3 TABLESPOONS CHOPPED MANGO CHUTNEY
2 TABLESPOONS PLAIN LOW-FAT YOGURT
2 TABLESPOONS REDUCED-CALORIE SOUR CREAM
1 TEASPOON CURRY POWDER
2 CUPS CHOPPED COOKED CHICKEN OR TURKEY (8 OUNCES)
½ CUP DICED UNPEELED APPLE (2 OUNCES)
½ CUP SHREDDED CARROT (2 OUNCES)

Method

1. Combine chutney, yogurt, sour cream, and curry powder in medium bowl.
2. Stir in chicken, apple, and carrot; mix well.
3. Chill at least 1 hour before serving.

Note: This salad is a perfect use for leftover roasted, broiled, or grilled chicken. Serve in whole wheat pita pockets for a delicious sandwich.

Marinated Red Onions

Yield: 2 cups (4 servings)
Serving Size: ½ cup
Exchanges:
Vegetable   1.0

Nutrient Content per Serving

CAL	33	Na	34 (mg)
PRO	1 (gm)	K	107 (mg)
Fat	1.8 (gm)	Fiber	2 (gm)
CHO	4 (gm)	Chol	0 (mg)

Ingredients

2 SMALL RED ONIONS, THINLY SLICED
¼ CUP RASPBERRY VINEGAR (PAGE 147)
1 TABLESPOON EXTRA-VIRGIN OLIVE OIL
½ TEASPOON SUGAR
⅛ TEASPOON SALT
4 LARGE LEAVES BOSTON LETTUCE
FRESHLY GROUND BLACK PEPPER

Method

1. Separate onions into rings; place in shallow glass dish or pie plate.
2. Combine vinegar, oil, sugar, and salt; pour over onions.
3. Cover and refrigerate at least 4 hours or overnight.
4. Serve on lettuce with pepper.

Roasted Pepper and Goat Cheese Salad

Yield: 2 cups (4 servings)
Serving Size: ½ cup
Exchanges:
Vegetable 1.0
Fat 1.0

Nutrient Content per Serving

CAL	62	*Na	52 (mg)
PRO	1 (gm)	K	151 (mg)
Fat	4.7 (gm)	Fiber	2.3 (gm)
CHO	5 (gm)	Chol	3 (mg)

*Add 33 mg if optional salt is used in the Balsamic Vinaigrette.

Ingredients

3 LARGE BELL PEPPERS, PREFERABLY 1 RED, 1 YEL-
   LOW, AND 1 ORANGE
¼ CUP FRESH BASIL LEAVES, CUT INTO THIN STRIPS
2 TABLESPOONS BALSAMIC VINAIGRETTE (PAGE 129)
2 TABLESPOONS FINELY CRUMBLED GOAT CHEESE
½ TEASPOON COARSELY GROUND BLACK PEPPER
   FRESH BASIL SPRIG (OPTIONAL)

Method

1. Cut peppers lengthwise into 4 quarters; discard seeds and membranes. Place skin side up on foil-lined cookie sheet.
2. Broil 2–3 inches from heat source until skin is charred and blackened, about 10–12 minutes.
3. Place peppers in paper bag; close and let stand until cool enough to handle. Peel and discard skin; cut peppers into 1-inch-wide strips and place in shallow serving dish.
4. Sprinkle evenly with basil; drizzle with vinaigrette. Sprinkle with goat cheese and black pepper. Serve at room temperature. Garnish with fresh basil sprig, if desired.

Note: This salad may be made ahead by combining peppers and vinaigrette. Cover and refrigerate up to 3 days. Bring to room temperature and finish assembly as directed above. This salad is a good accompaniment to grilled meats and poultry.

Asparagus, Leek, and Red Pepper Salad

Yield: 4 servings
Serving Size: ¼ recipe
Exchanges:
Vegetable   1.0
Fat   1.0

Nutrient Content per Serving

CAL	71	Na	21 (mg)
PRO	1 (gm)	K	164 (mg)
Fat	5.4 (gm)	Fiber	2 (gm)
CHO	6 (gm)	Chol	0 (mg)

Ingredients

> 6 OUNCES FRESH ASPARAGUS, TRIMMED AND CUT INTO 1-INCH PIECES
> 1 LARGE LEEK, WHITE PART PLUS 1 INCH LIGHT GREEN, THINLY SLICED INTO RINGS
> 1 SMALL RED BELL PEPPER, CUT INTO SHORT, THIN STRIPS (1 CUP)
> 1½ TABLESPOONS RED WINE VINEGAR
> 1 TEASPOON DIJON MUSTARD
> ½ TEASPOON DRIED TARRAGON
> ¼ TEASPOON FRESHLY GROUND BLACK PEPPER
> 1½ TABLESPOONS EXTRA-VIRGIN OLIVE OIL
> RADICCHIO LEAVES (OPTIONAL)

Method

1. Blanch asparagus and leeks in boiling water 3–4 minutes or just until tender. Rinse with cold water and drain well. Transfer to medium bowl; toss with red pepper.
2. Combine vinegar, mustard, tarragon, and pepper. Whisk in oil until well blended. Pour over asparagus mixture. Serve at room temperature or chilled on radicchio leaves, if desired.

Method-Microwave

1. Place asparagus and leeks in microwave-safe casserole dish. Cover with vented plastic wrap. Cook on high power 2–3 minutes or just until tender. Rinse with cold water and drain well. Transfer to medium bowl; toss with red pepper.
2. Proceed as directed above in step 2.

Note: This salad travels well and looks pretty on a buffet table long after others have wilted. Bring it to your next potluck dinner and get ready for the compliments.

Southwestern Orange and Jicama Salad

Yield: 3 cups (6 servings)
Serving Size: ½ cup
Exchanges:
Fruit   0.5
Fat   0.5

Nutrient Content per Serving

CAL	58	Na	22 (mg)
PRO	1 (gm)	K	148 (mg)
Fat	2.6 (gm)	Fiber	1 (gm)
CHO	9 (gm)	Chol	0 (mg)

Ingredients

    2 MEDIUM NAVEL ORANGES (1 POUND)
    1 CUP SHORT, THIN JICAMA STRIPS (4 OUNCES)
    2 TABLESPOONS PREPARED HOT SALSA OR PICANTE
      SAUCE
    1 TABLESPOON SUNFLOWER OR CORN OIL
    1 TABLESPOON CIDER VINEGAR
    2 TABLESPOONS CHOPPED CILANTRO (OPTIONAL)

Method

1. Peel oranges, separate into sections, and slice each section in half crosswise. Combine oranges and jicama in medium bowl.
2. Combine remaining ingredients except cilantro; mix well. Pour over orange mixture. Chill at least 1 hour before serving. Sprinkle with cilantro, if desired.

Note: Jicama may be considered a "new" vegetable to many. This recipe calls for approximately half a small jicama. It should be peeled with a paring knife and cut into strips for most uses.

Corn Relish Salad

Yield: 2½ cups (5 servings)
Serving Size: ½ cup
Exchanges:
Starch/Bread   1.0
Fat   1.0

Nutrient Content per Serving

CAL	112	*Na	6 (mg)
PRO	2 (gm)	K	189 (mg)
Fat	5.6 (gm)	Fiber	4 (gm)
CHO	16 (gm)	Chol	0 (mg)

*Add 107 mg if optional salt is added.

Ingredients

1 10-OUNCE PACKAGE FROZEN WHOLE KERNEL CORN, THAWED, OR 2 CUPS FRESH KERNELS
1 CUP DICED RED OR ORANGE BELL PEPPER (4 OUNCES)
⅓ CUP SLICED GREEN ONIONS WITH TOPS (½ OUNCE)
⅓ CUP CHOPPED FRESH CILANTRO
2 TABLESPOONS FRESH LIME JUICE
2 TABLESPOONS EXTRA-VIRGIN OLIVE OIL
¼–½ TEASPOON HOT PEPPER SAUCE, AS DESIRED
¼ TEASPOON SALT (OPTIONAL)
5 LARGE RED LEAF LETTUCE LEAVES

Method

1. Combine corn, bell peppers, onions, and cilantro in medium bowl.
2. Whisk together lime juice, oil, pepper sauce, and salt, if desired; pour over corn mixture. Toss well, cover, and chill at least 1 hour. Serve on lettuce leaves.

Note: This salad is particularly good when sweet corn is in season. Steam or boil 3–4 large ears of corn; cool and cut kernels from cobs as a substitute for frozen corn.

Best Ever Coleslaw

Yield: 4 cups (8 servings)   Nutrient Content per Serving
Serving Size: ½ cup

Serving Size: ½ cup

CAL	93	Na	140 (mg)
PRO	2 (gm)	K	183 (mg)
Fat	5.6 (gm)	Fiber	2 (gm)
CHO	10 (gm)	Chol	6 (mg)

Exchanges:
Vegetable   2.0
Fat   1.0

Ingredients

    1 SMALL OR ½ LARGE HEAD CABBAGE (1½ POUNDS)
    ½ CUP REDUCED-CALORIE MAYONNAISE
    ½ CUP REDUCED-CALORIE SOUR CREAM
    2 TABLESPOONS SUGAR
    2 TABLESPOONS PREPARED HORSERADISH
    1 TABLESPOON FRESH LEMON JUICE
    ¼ TEASPOON DRY MUSTARD
    ⅛ TEASPOON CAYENNE (GROUND RED) PEPPER
    ⅛ TEASPOON EACH GARLIC POWDER, ONION POW-
      DER, AND CELERY SALT

Method

1. Chop cabbage into large chunks. Place several chunks in food processor fitted with steel blade. Do not overfill processor. Chop fine using on/off turns; transfer to large bowl. Repeat with remaining cabbage, Do not wash bowl of food processor.
2. Add remaining ingredients to food processor; process until well combined. Pour over cabbage; cover and refrigerate at least 8 hours or overnight.

Note: The flavor of this coleslaw improves upon standing. Adjust seasoning, if desired, after 8 hours or overnight. The celery salt is the key ingredient. It will keep tightly covered and refrigerated up to 6 days. Stir well before serving. A must for the all-American barbecue table!

Fresh Tomato Aspic

Yield: 6 servings
Serving Size: ⅙ recipe
Exchanges:
Vegetable   1.0

Nutrient Content per Serving

CAL	34	*Na	42 (mg)
PRO	2 (gm)	K	207 (mg)
Fat	1.7 (gm)	Fiber	1 (gm)
CHO	4 (gm)	Chol	2 (mg)

*Add 178 mg if optional salt is used.

Ingredients

    2 CUPS PEELED, SEEDED, AND FINELY CHOPPED
      FRESH TOMATOES
    1 ENVELOPE UNFLAVORED GELATIN
    2 TEASPOONS EXTRA-VIRGIN BALSAMIC OR RED
      WINE VINEGAR
    ¼ CUP VERY FINELY CHOPPED CELERY LEAVES
    ½ TEASPOON SALT (OPTIONAL)
    ¼ TEASPOON FRESHLY GROUND BLACK PEPPER
    6 LETTUCE LEAVES
    2 TABLESPOONS REDUCED-CALORIE MAYONNAISE

Method

1. Place 1 cup tomatoes in small saucepan; sprinkle with gelatin. Bring just to a boil over medium heat, stirring constantly, until gelatin is dissolved.
2. Remove from heat; stir in remaining tomatoes, vinegar, celery leaves, salt (if desired), and pepper. Mix well and pour into a 7-by-3-inch nonstick loaf pan.
3. Cover and refrigerate until firm or overnight. Unmold; slice and place on lettuce. Dollop each serving with 1 teaspoon reduced-calorie mayonnaise.

Note: This recipe is a Southern treat from the 50s that is too good to leave in the cookbook archives. Fresh parsley may be substituted for the celery leaves.

Greek Chick-Pea Salad

Yield: 3 cups (6 servings)
Serving Size: ½ cup
Exchanges:
Starch/Bread   1.0
Vegetable   1.0
Fat   1.0

Nutrient Content per Serving

CAL	146	Na	130 (mg)
PRO	6 (gm)	K	249 (mg)
Fat	6.9 (gm)	Fiber	3 (gm)
CHO	17 (gm)	Chol	4 (mg)

Ingredients

    1 CAN (ABOUT 16 OUNCES) GARBANZO BEANS (CHICK-
    PEAS), RINSED AND DRAINED
    1 SMALL TOMATO, SEEDED AND CHOPPED (4 OUNCES,
    1 CUP)
    ½ CUP DICED UNPEELED CUCUMBER (2 OUNCES)
    ⅓ CUP (2 MEDIUM) SLICED GREEN ONIONS (1 OUNCE)
    ¼ CUP COARSELY CHOPPED ITALIAN PARSLEY
    2 TABLESPOONS RED WINE VINEGAR
    2 TABLESPOONS EXTRA-VIRGIN OLIVE OIL
    ¼ CUP (1 OUNCE) CRUMBLED FETA CHEESE
    FRESHLY GROUND BLACK PEPPER

Method

1. Combine beans, tomato, cucumber, onions, and parsley in medium bowl.
2. Whisk together vinegar and oil; pour over bean mixture. Toss well. Just before serving, sprinkle with cheese; serve with pepper.

Greek-Style Tossed Salad

		Nutrient Content per Serving			
Yield: 4 servings					
Serving Size: ¼ recipe		CAL	92	Na	48 (mg)
Exchanges:		PRO	2 (gm)	K	272 (mg)
Vegetable	1.0	Fat	7.7 (gm)	Fiber	1.4 (gm)
Fat	1.5	CHO	5 (gm)	Chol	3 (mg)

Ingredients

- 2 CUPS TORN ROMAINE LETTUCE
- 1 LARGE TOMATO, SEEDED AND CUT INTO LARGE CHUNKS
- 1 SMALL CUCUMBER, SCORED BUT UNPEELED, THINLY SLICED
- 2 TABLESPOONS EXTRA-VIRGIN OLIVE OIL
- 1 TABLESPOON FRESH LEMON JUICE
- 1 TABLESPOON RED WINE VINEGAR
- 1 TABLESPOON CHOPPED FRESH MARJORAM OR OREGANO OR 1 TEASPOON DRIED MARJORAM OR OREGANO
- 1 CLOVE GARLIC, MINCED
- ¼ TEASPOON FRESHLY GROUND BLACK PEPPER
- 2 TABLESPOONS CRUMBLED FETA OR GOAT CHEESE

Method

1. Toss romaine, tomato, and cucumber in large serving bowl.
2. Whisk together oil, lemon juice, vinegar, marjoram, garlic, and pepper. Toss with romaine mixture; sprinkle with cheese.

Pear, Blue Cheese, and Endive Salad

Yield: 2 servings	Nutrient Content per Serving		
Serving Size: ½ recipe	CAL 149	Na	144 (mg)
Exchanges:	PRO 3 (gm)	K	331 (mg)
Fruit 1.0	Fat 9.4 (gm)	Fiber	4 (gm)
Fat 2.0	CHO 16 (gm)	Chol	5 (mg)

Ingredients

- 1 TABLESPOON WALNUT OIL OR EXTRA-VIRGIN OLIVE OIL
- 1 TABLESPOON RASPBERRY OR BALSAMIC VINEGAR
- 1 TEASPOON DIJON MUSTARD
- ¼ TEASPOON SUGAR
- 2 LARGE LEAVES RED LEAF LETTUCE
- 1 RIPE MEDIUM PEAR, PREFERABLY BOSC
- 1 SMALL HEAD FRESH BELGIAN ENDIVE, SEPARATED INTO LEAVES
- 2 TABLESPOONS CRUMBLED BLUE CHEESE (½ OUNCE) FRESHLY GROUND BLACK PEPPER

Method

1. Whisk together oil, vinegar, mustard, and sugar.
2. Line 2 salad plates with lettuce leaves. Peel, core, and slice pear lengthwise into ½-inch slices.
3. Alternately fan pear slices with endive leaves over lettuce leaves. Sprinkle with cheese.
4. Drizzle dressing evenly over salads; serve with pepper.

Note: This salad typifies a perfect marriage of tart and sweet. Serve it as a dramatic first course at an intimate dinner party.

Tabbouli Salad

Yield: 3 cups (6 servings)	Nutrient Content per Serving			
Serving Size: ½ cup	CAL	131	Na	14 (mg)
Exchanges:	PRO	3 (gm)	K	145 (mg)
Starch/Bread 1.0	Fat	5.1 (gm)	Fiber	1 (gm)
Fat 1.0	CHO	19 (gm)	Chol	0 (mg)

Ingredients

2 TABLESPOONS EXTRA-VIRGIN OLIVE OIL
¾ CUP BULGUR WHEAT
¾ CUP REDUCED-SODIUM CHICKEN BROTH
¼ CUP FRESH LEMON JUICE (OR 2 TABLESPOONS LEMON JUICE AND 2 TABLESPOONS LIME JUICE)
¼ TEASPOON SALT (OPTIONAL)
½ TEASPOON FRESHLY GROUND BLACK PEPPER
2 TABLESPOONS CHOPPED FRESH MINT
1 LARGE TOMATO, SEEDED AND CHOPPED (8 OUNCES, 1½ CUPS)
⅓ CUP (2 MEDIUM) THINLY SLICED GREEN ONIONS (1 OUNCE)
MINT LEAVES (OPTIONAL)

Method

1. Heat 1 tablespoon oil in 10-inch skillet over medium-high heat. Add the bulgur and toss until coated with oil, about 1 minute.
2. Add broth and bring to a boil. Remove from heat. Let stand covered until all the liquid is absorbed, about 1 hour.
3. Combine remaining 1 tablespoon oil, lemon juice, salt (if desired), and pepper in medium bowl. Add bulgur, mint, tomato, and green onions; toss. Garnish with mint leaves, if desired; serve at room temperature or chill.

Note: This salad is perfect for summer dining when tomatoes and mint are in season. If fresh mint is unavailable, use 2 teaspoons dried mint plus 2 tablespoons chopped parsley.

Fresh mint is easy to grow in a sunny, well-drained location, but keep it in a pot to inhibit its tendency to take over the garden. Transfer to a sunny window indoors during cooler months.

Mild Oriental Flavored Oil

Yield: 5 tablespoons (10 servings)
Serving Size: 1½ teaspoons
Exchanges:
Fat   1.5

Nutrient Content per Serving			
CAL	66	Na	0 (mg)
PRO	0 (gm)	K	0 (mg)
Fat	7.5 (gm)	Fiber	0 (gm)
CHO	0 (gm)	Chol	0 (mg)

Ingredients

⅓ CUP PEANUT OIL
6 SLICES FRESH GINGERROOT, CUT ⅛ INCH THICK (1 OUNCE)
4 CLOVES GARLIC, PEELED AND HALVED
½ TEASPOON RED PEPPER FLAKES

Method

1. Combine oil and ginger in small saucepan. Heat over medium heat until bubbly.
2. Remove from heat; add garlic and pepper flakes. Let stand at room temperature 4–6 hours.
3. Strain oil; discard solids. Use to stir-fry vegetables or in salads such as Korean Noodle Salad (pages 260–261). Oil will keep refrigerated up to 3 months.

Note: Any infused oil is subject to bacterial growth if not kept refrigerated. The oil may solidify, but will melt quickly at room temperature.

Salad of Shrimp and Asparagus

Yield: 2 servings
Serving Size: ½ recipe
Exchanges:
Meat, lean 2.0
Vegetable 1.0
Fat 2.0

Nutrient Content per Serving

CAL	216	Na	201 (mg)
PRO	15 (gm)	K	582 (mg)
Fat	14.8 (gm)	Fiber	3.6 (gm)
CHO	8 (gm)	Chol	111 (mg)

Ingredients

2 TABLESPOONS WHITE WINE VINEGAR
2 TABLESPOONS EXTRA-VIRGIN OLIVE OIL
2 TABLESPOONS DIJON-STYLE MUSTARD
2 TEASPOONS CHOPPED FRESH TARRAGON OR ½ TEASPOON DRIED TARRAGON LEAVES, CRUSHED
6 LARGE BOSTON LETTUCE LEAVES (3 OUNCES)
8 LARGE ASPARAGUS SPEARS, COOKED CRISP-TENDER, CHILLED
¼ POUND SMALL COOKED SHELLED SHRIMP (BAY SHRIMP), THAWED IF FROZEN
2 TABLESPOONS FINELY DICED RED BELL PEPPER FRESHLY GROUND BLACK PEPPER

Method

1. Combine vinegar, oil, mustard, and tarragon; whisk until smooth and slightly thickened. Refrigerate until serving.
2. Arrange 3 lettuce leaves on each of 2 salad plates. Top with asparagus and shrimp. Drizzle with dressing; sprinkle with red pepper. Serve with pepper.

Chinese Slaw

Yield: 4 servings	Nutrient Content per Serving		
Serving Size: ¼ recipe	CAL	58	Na	157 (mg)
Exchanges:	PRO	1 (gm)	K	193 (mg)
Vegetable	1.0	Fat	4.3 (gm)	Fiber	3.4 (gm)
Fat	1.0	CHO	5 (gm)	Chol	0 (mg)

Ingredients

 2 CUPS SHREDDED NAPA (CHINESE) CABBAGE OR
   GREEN CABBAGE
 1 CUP SHREDDED RED CABBAGE
 ½ CUP SLICED GREEN ONIONS
 ½ CUP COARSELY CHOPPED CILANTRO OR PARSLEY
 1 TABLESPOON ORIENTAL SESAME OIL
 1 TABLESPOON DRY SHERRY
 1 TABLESPOON REDUCED-SODIUM SOY SAUCE
 1 TABLESPOON RICE WINE VINEGAR OR WHITE WINE
   VINEGAR
 1 CLOVE GARLIC, MINCED
 ¼ TEASPOON CRUSHED SZECHUAN PEPPERCORNS
   OR RED PEPPER FLAKES
 2 TEASPOONS TOASTED SESAME SEEDS

Method

1. Combine cabbages, onions, and cilantro in large serving bowl.
2. Whisk together remaining ingredients except sesame seeds; pour over cabbage mixture. Toss well. Sprinkle with sesame seeds.

Garlic-Buttermilk Dressing

Yield: 6 tablespoons
Serving Size: 1 tablespoon
Exchanges:
Fat   1.0

Nutrient Content per Serving

CAL	44	Na	100 (mg)
PRO	0 (gm)	K	17 (mg)
Fat	4.6 (gm)	Fiber	0 (gm)
CHO	1 (gm)	Chol	0 (mg)

Ingredients

¼ CUP LOW-FAT BUTTERMILK
2 TABLESPOONS OLIVE OIL
1 SMALL CLOVE GARLIC, MINCED
½ TEASPOON FRESHLY GROUND BLACK PEPPER
¼ TEASPOON SALT

Method

1. Whisk together all ingredients.

Variation: For herbed garlic-buttermilk dressing, add 1 table-spoon chopped fresh tarragon, dill, thyme, rosemary, oregano, basil, or parsley or 1 teaspoon dried.

Thousand Island Dressing

Yield: ¾ cup (12 servings)
Serving Size: 1 tablespoon
Exchanges:
Fat   0.5

Nutrient Content per Serving

CAL	34	Na	69 (mg)
PRO	0 (gm)	K	19 (mg)
Fat	3.1 (gm)	Fiber	0 (gm)
CHO	2 (gm)	Chol	4 (mg)

Ingredients

½ CUP REDUCED-CALORIE MAYONNAISE
¼ CUP NO-SALT-ADDED CHILI SAUCE
1 TABLESPOON SWEET PICKLE RELISH
¼ TEASPOON RED PEPPER SAUCE

Method

1. Combine all ingredients; chill until ready to serve (up to 5 days).

Raspberry Vinegar

Yield: 2 cups (16 servings)
Serving Size: 1 tablespoon

Nutrient Content per Serving

CAL	2	Na	0 (mg)
PRO	0 (gm)	K	15 (mg)
Fat	0 (gm)	Fiber	0 (gm)
CHO	1 (gm)	Chol	0 (mg)

Ingredients

    2 CUPS WHITE WINE VINEGAR
    1 CUP FRESH RASPBERRIES

Method

1. Combine vinegar and raspberries in clean glass jar. Cover tightly and let stand in cool dry place away from direct light for 2 weeks.
2. Strain out berries using fine strainer. Let stand in strainer to drain, but do not push on berries. Transfer strained vinegar to sterilized bottles; cover tightly. Store in cool dry place away from direct light. Vinegar will keep for up to 6 months.

Variation: To make herbed vinegar, use favorite herb sprigs (such as basil, tarragon, rosemary, or thyme—not chives), cleaned but not cut up. See page 146. Cover all surfaces with white or red wine vinegar and proceed as directed above.

For garlic vinegar, thread peeled garlic cloves onto wooden skewers and cover surfaces with white or red wine vinegar and proceed as directed above.

Note: Unlike flavored oils, flavored vinegars may be kept at room temperature without concern for bacterial growth due to their acid content.

New Potato and Green Bean Salad

Yield: 8 servings
Serving Size: ⅛ recipe
Exchanges:
Starch/Bread   1.0
Fat   1.0

Nutrient Content per Serving

CAL	123	Na	51 (mg)
PRO	2 (gm)	K	291 (mg)
Fat	7.1 (gm)	Fiber	2.2 (gm)
CHO	14 (gm)	Chol	0 (mg)

Ingredients

1 POUND NEW POTATOES,UNPEELED
8 OUNCES GREEN OR WAX BEANS, CUT INTO 1-INCH PIECES (2 CUPS)
¼ CUP OLIVE OIL
2 TABLESPOONS DIJON MUSTARD OR TARRAGON DI-JON MUSTARD
2 TABLESPOONS CIDER VINEGAR
2 TABLESPOONS CHOPPED FRESH CHIVES OR GREEN ONION TOPS
2 TABLESPOONS CRUMBLED ROQUEFORT OR BLUE CHEESE (OPTIONAL)

Method

1. Cook potatoes in boiling water 6 minutes. Add beans; continue to boil until potatoes are tender and beans are crisp-tender, about 4–6 minutes longer. Drain. Cut potatoes into bite-size pieces; transfer to large bowl with beans.
2. Whisk together oil, mustard, and vinegar; pour over warm potatoes and beans. Cover and refrigerate at least 4 hours. Just before serving, stir in chives and cheese, if desired.

Method-Microwave

1. Pierce each potato once with a fork. Place on paper towel in microwave oven and cook on high power 7–8 minutes or until almost tender. Let stand 5 minutes; cut into bite-size pieces.

2. Place beans in large microwave-safe serving bowl. Cover with vented plastic wrap. Cook on high power 2–3 minutes or until crisp-tender. Let stand 5 minutes; drain. Add potatoes to beans. Proceed as in step 2 above.

Note: This salad is perfect for a potluck get-together or block party. It may be served at room temperature as well as chilled, and is a refreshing change from heavy mayonnaise-based potato salads.

Fresh Mushroom Salad Mimosa

Yield: 4 servings		Nutrient Content per Serving		
Serving Size: ¼ recipe		CAL	54	Na	85 (mg)
Exchanges:		PRO	2 (gm)	K	263 (mg)
Vegetable	1.0	Fat	3.4 (gm)	Fiber	1.7 (gm)
Fat	0.5	CHO	5 (gm)	Chol	4 (mg)

Ingredients

    8 OUNCES FRESH MUSHROOMS, SLICED (ABOUT 3
    CUPS)
    ¼ CUP THOUSAND ISLAND DRESSING (PAGES 146–147)
    4 LARGE BOSTON OR RED LEAF LETTUCE LEAVES
    1 HARD-COOKED EGG WHITE, MINCED
    2 TABLESPOONS CHOPPED CHIVES OR PARSLEY
    FRESHLY GROUND BLACK PEPPER

Method

1. Toss mushrooms with dressing; mix well.
2. Line 4 serving plates with lettuce; divide mushroom mixture over lettuce. Sprinkle with egg white and chives. Serve with pepper.

Bay Area Rice Salad

		Nutrient Content per Serving			
Yield: 6 cups (6 servings)					
Serving Size: 1 cup		CAL	186	Na	161 (mg)
Exchanges:		PRO	10 (gm)	K	167 (mg)
Starch/Bread	1.5	Fat	4.3 (gm)	Fiber	1.8 (gm)
Meat, lean	1.0	CHO	26 (gm)	Chol	19 (mg)
Vegetable	1.0				

Ingredients

- 2 CUPS CHILLED COOKED WHITE RICE
- 1 CUP CHILLED COOKED WILD RICE
- 1 CUP SMOKED MUSSELS OR SMOKED BAY SCALLOPS (6 OUNCES)*
- ½ CUP DICED RED BELL PEPPER
- ½ CUP DICED YELLOW OR GREEN BELL PEPPER
- ½ CUP DICED UNPEELED AND SEEDED CUCUMBER
- 3 TABLESPOONS REDUCED-CALORIE MAYONNAISE
- 3 TABLESPOONS REDUCED-CALORIE SOUR CREAM
- 1 TABLESPOON CHOPPED FRESH DILL OR 1 TEASPOON DRIED DILL WEED
- 2 TEASPOONS LEMON JUICE
- ¼ TEASPOON FRESHLY GROUND BLACK PEPPER

Method

1. Combine rices, mussels, peppers, and cucumbers in large bowl. Combine remaining ingredients; mix well. Toss with rice mixture. Serve immediately or chill. Let stand at room temperature 30 minutes before serving.

*Smoked mussels or bay scallops are available in specialty fish markets. Poached mussels or bay scallops may be substituted.

Carrot Salad with Dill

Yield: 2⅔ cups (4 servings)
Serving Size: ¼ recipe
Exchanges:
Vegetable   2.0
Fat   1.0

Nutrient Content per Serving

CAL	95	*Na	55 (mg)
PRO	1 (gm)	K	220 (mg)
Fat	5.8 (gm)	Fiber	3.1 (gm)
CHO	11 (gm)	Chol	0 (mg)

*Add 267 mg if optional salt is used.

Ingredients

   3 CUPS THINLY SLICED CARROTS (12 OUNCES)
   ½ CUP FINELY CHOPPED RED OR SWEET WHITE
      ONION (2 OUNCES)
1½ TABLESPOONS VEGETABLE OIL
   1 TABLESPOON SHERRY OR CHAMPAGNE VINEGAR
   1 TABLESPOON CHOPPED FRESH DILL OR 1 TEASPOON
      DRIED DILL WEED
   ½ TEASPOON SUGAR
   ½ TEASPOON SALT (OPTIONAL)
      FRESHLY GROUND BLACK PEPPER

Method

1. Cook carrots in boiling water or steamer until crisp-tender, about 6–8 minutes. Rinse with cold water; drain well.
2. Combine carrots and onion in medium bowl. Combine oil, vinegar, dill, sugar, and salt, if desired; mix well. Toss with carrot mixture. Chill. Serve with pepper.

Method-Microwave

1. Place carrots in shallow microwave-safe casserole dish. Cover with vented plastic wrap. Cook on high power 4–6 minutes or until crisp-tender. Rinse with cold water; drain well.
2. Continue as directed in step 2 above.

Note: This salad is a great source of vitamin A.

Golden Gate Bean Salad

Yield: 2 cups (4 servings)
Serving Size: ½ cup
Exchanges:

		Nutrient Content per Serving			
		CAL	176	*Na	149 (mg)
		PRO	8 (gm)	K	504 (mg)
Starch/Bread	1.0	Fat	5.8 (gm)	Fiber	7.2 (gm)
Vegetable	2.0	CHO	24 (gm)	Chol	0 (mg)
Fat	1.0				

*Add 49 mg if optional salt is used in the Balsamic Vinaigrette.

Ingredients

1 19-OUNCE CAN CANNELLINI BEANS, RINSED AND DRAINED*
2 LARGE RED BELL PEPPERS, ROASTED, PEELED, AND CUT INTO SHORT, THIN STRIPS
3 TABLESPOONS BALSAMIC VINAIGRETTE (PAGE 129)
¼ CUP COARSELY CHOPPED FRESH BASIL, CILANTRO OR ITALIAN PARSLEY LEAVES
CRACKED BLACK PEPPER

Method

1. Combine beans, peppers, and vinaigrette; toss. Chill until serving time. Just before serving, stir in cilantro; sprinkle with pepper to taste. Serve chilled or at room temperature.

*If cannellini beans are not available, substitute 1 16-ounce can white Great Northern beans.

Marinated Crisp Vegetable Salad

Yield: 6 servings	Nutrient Content per Serving		
Serving Size: ⅙ recipe	CAL 105	Na	45 (mg)
Exchanges:	PRO 1 (gm)	K	229 (mg)
Vegetable 1.0	Fat 9.3 (gm)	Fiber	2.2 (gm)
Fat 2.0	CHO 6 (gm)	Chol	0 (mg)

Ingredients

- 1 CUP DIAGONALLY SLICED CARROTS
- 1 CUP BROCCOLI FLORETS
- 1 CUP CAULIFLOWERETS
- 1 RED BELL PEPPER, CUT INTO 1-INCH PIECES
- ⅓ CUP TARRAGON OR WHITE WINE VINEGAR
- ¼ CUP OLIVE OIL
- 1 TABLESPOON COUNTRY-STYLE OR TARRAGON DI-
  JON MUSTARD
- ½ TEASPOON FRESHLY GROUND BLACK PEPPER

Method

1. Bring a large saucepan of water to a boil. Drop carrots, broccoli, and cauliflower into water. Return to a boil; boil 30–60
   seconds so vegetables remain very crisp. Drain and rinse with
   cold water. Drain well and transfer to large bowl.
2. Add red pepper. Combine vinegar, oil, mustard, and pepper.
   Toss with vegetables. Refrigerate, covered, until serving time.

Method-Microwave

1. Place carrots, broccoli, and cauliflower in shallow microwave-
   safe casserole dish. Cover with vented plastic wrap. Cook on
   high power 3–4 minutes. (Vegetables will be very crisp.) Rinse
   with cold water until cooled. Drain and transfer to large bowl.
2. Continue as directed in step 2 above.

Breads, Muffins, and Biscuits

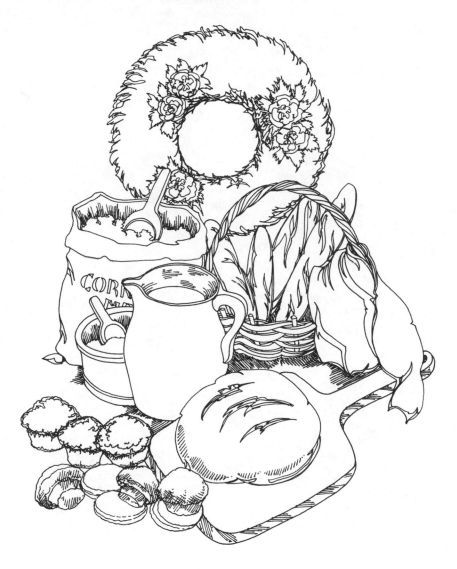

Whole Wheat Yogurt Pancakes

Yield: 12 pancakes (4 servings)		Nutrient Content per Serving			
Serving Size: 3 pancakes		CAL	213	Na	353 (mg)
Exchanges:		PRO	9 (gm)	K	316 (mg)
Starch/Bread	2.0	Fat	1.6 (gm)	Fiber	2.9 (gm)
Fruit	1.0	CHO	43 (gm)	*Chol	4 (mg)

*Add 69 mg if whole egg is used.

Ingredients

      1 CUP WHOLE WHEAT FLOUR
      2 TEASPOONS SUGAR
      1 TEASPOON BAKING POWDER
      ½ TEASPOON BAKING SODA
      ⅛ TEASPOON SALT
      ¼ CUP EGG SUBSTITUTE OR 1 EGG
      ½ CUP PLAIN LOW-FAT YOGURT
      1 CUP LOW-FAT BUTTERMILK
      ¼ CUP JAM, MARMALADE, OR CONSERVE

Method

1. Combine flour, sugar, baking powder, soda, and salt.
2. Beat egg substitute with yogurt; add buttermilk. Add to dry ingredients; mix just until dry ingredients are moistened. Batter may be lumpy.
3. Heat large nonstick skillet or griddle over medium heat. Pour ¼ cup batter for each pancake; cook until browned, about 2 minutes. Turn and cook until browned, about 1 minute. Serve with preserves.

Note: Because of its sugar content, this recipe should be for occasional use only. Pancakes may be wrapped securely and frozen up to 3 months. To reheat, wrap in foil and place in 350°F oven or toaster oven until hot, or wrap in paper towel and microwave on high power about 45 seconds per pancake.

Savory Pancake Puff

Yield: 4 servings

Serving Size: ¼ pancake puff

Exchanges:

Starch/Bread 1.0

Fat 1.0

Nutrient Content per Serving

CAL	126	Na	264 (mg)
PRO	6 (gm)	K	164 (mg)
Fat	6 (gm)	Fiber	0.8 (gm)
CHO	12 (gm)	*Chol	0 (mg)

*Add 138 mg if whole eggs are used.

Ingredients

    NONSTICK COOKING SPRAY
1 SMALL ONION, FINELY CHOPPED
2 TABLESPOONS MARGARINE
1 TABLESPOON FRESH CHOPPED ROSEMARY OR 1
    TEASPOON CRUSHED DRIED ROSEMARY
¾ CUP SKIM MILK
⅓ CUP ALL-PURPOSE FLOUR
¼ TEASPOON SALT
½ CUP EGG SUBSTITUTE OR 2 EGGS

Method

1. Preheat oven to 400°F. Coat inside of 10-inch glass pie plate with cooking spray.
2. Sauté onion in margarine 3 minutes. Stir in rosemary; cook 1 minute more.
3. Combine remaining ingredients in blender container or food processor fitted with steel blade. Blend or process until smooth. Add onion mixture. Pour into pie plate. Bake until puffed and golden brown, 25–30 minutes. Cut into 4 wedges; serve warm.

Northern-Style Double Corn Muffins

Yield: 1 dozen muffins
Serving Size: 1 muffin
Exchanges:
Starch/Bread   1.0
Fat   0.5

Nutrient Content per Serving	with egg substitute	with whole egg
CAL	107	111
PRO	3 (gm)	3 (gm)
Fat	2.3 (gm)	2.8 (gm)
CHO	19 (gm)	19 (gm)
Na	137 (mg)	136 (mg)
K	78 (mg)	77 (mg)
Fiber	2 (gm)	2 (gm)
Chol	1 (mg)	24 (mg)

Ingredients

- 1 CUP YELLOW OR WHITE CORNMEAL
- ½ CUP FLOUR
- 1 TABLESPOON GRANULATED FRUCTOSE OR SUGAR (OPTIONAL)
- 2 TEASPOONS BAKING POWDER
- ½ TEASPOON BAKING SODA
- 1 CUP FROZEN CORN KERNELS, THAWED (4 OUNCES)
- 1 CUP LOW-FAT BUTTERMILK
- ¼ CUP EGG SUBSTITUTE OR 1 EGG, BEATEN
- 2 TABLESPOONS MARGARINE, MELTED

Method

1. Combine cornmeal, flour, fructose, baking powder, and baking soda in medium bowl. Stir in corn.
2. Add buttermilk, egg substitute, and margarine; mix just until dry ingredients are moistened.
3. Line medium-sized muffin cups with paper liners; fill ¾ full with batter.
4. Bake in 400°F oven 15 minutes. Serve warm.

Note: Muffins may be kept frozen up to 3 months. To reheat each frozen muffin, wrap in paper towel and cook on high power in microwave about 30 seconds, or wrap in foil and heat in 350°F oven about 15 minutes.

Applesauce-Raisin Muffins

Yield: 12 muffins
Serving Size: 1 muffin
Exchanges:
Starch/Bread   1.5

Nutrient Content per Serving		
	with egg substitute	with whole egg
CAL	130	139
PRO	4 (gm)	4.1 (gm)
Fat	2.4 (gm)	3.3 (gm)
CHO	24 (gm)	23.9 (gm)
Na	189 (mg)	188 (mg)
K	150 (mg)	146 (mg)
Fiber	2 (gm)	1.8 (gm)
Chol	1 (mg)	46 (mg)

Ingredients

1 CUP ALL-PURPOSE FLOUR
¾ CUP WHOLE WHEAT FLOUR
2 TABLESPOONS BROWN SUGAR
2 TEASPOONS BAKING POWDER
1 TEASPOON CINNAMON
½ TEASPOON NUTMEG
½ TEASPOON GROUND CLOVES
½ TEASPOON BAKING SODA
¼ TEASPOON SALT
½ CUP RAISINS
½ CUP EGG SUBSTITUTE OR 2 EGGS
¾ CUP UNSWEETENED APPLESAUCE
1 CUP LOW-FAT BUTTERMILK
2 TABLESPOONS CORN OR SAFFLOWER OIL

Method

1. Preheat oven to 400°F. Line 12 medium muffin cups with paper liners; set aside.
2. Combine flours, sugar, baking powder, spices, soda, and salt in large bowl. Stir in raisins.
3. Combine remaining ingredients; stir into dry ingredients, mixing just until moistened.
4. Fill muffin cups almost full. Bake 25–30 minutes or until wooden pick inserted in center comes out clean.
5. Cool 15 minutes in tin on wire rack; serve warm.

Cheese and Basil Scones

Yield: 12 scones
Serving Size: 1 scone
Exchanges:
Starch/Bread 1.0
Fat 1.0

Nutrient Content per Serving

CAL	126	Na	128 (mg)
PRO	4 (gm)	K	49 (mg)
Fat	4.1 (gm)	Fiber	1 (gm)
CHO	18 (gm)	*Chol	2 (mg)

*Add 23 mg if whole egg is used.

Ingredients

2 CUPS FLOUR
¼ CUP (1 OUNCE) FRESHLY GRATED PARMESAN OR ROMANO CHEESE
2 TEASPOONS BAKING POWDER
½ TEASPOON BAKING SODA
2 TABLESPOONS CHOPPED FRESH BASIL LEAVES OR 2 TEASPOONS DRIED BASIL
¼ TEASPOON FRESHLY GROUND BLACK PEPPER
⅔ CUP LOW-FAT BUTTERMILK
3 TABLESPOONS GOOD-QUALITY OLIVE OIL
NONSTICK VEGETABLE SPRAY
1 TABLESPOON EGG SUBSTITUTE OR 1 EGG, BEATEN (OPTIONAL)

Method

1. Preheat oven to 450°F.
2. Combine flour, cheese, baking powder, soda, basil, and pepper in medium bowl.
3. Add buttermilk and oil; mix only until dry ingredients are moistened. Divide dough into 2 balls. Knead gently 3 times on floured surface.
4. Spray cookie sheet with vegetable spray. Pat dough into 2 circles 7–8 inches in diameter. With sharp knife, score each disk (¼ inch deep) into 6 wedges, but do not cut through.
5. Brush with egg substitute, if desired, to glaze. Bake 10–12 minutes or until golden brown. Cut into wedges and serve warm or at room temperature.

Note: Scones may be wrapped securely and frozen up to 3 months. Reheat in 350°F oven uncovered 10 minutes, or wrap each scone in a paper towel and cook on high power in microwave oven 30–40 seconds.

Orange-Currant Oat-Bran Muffins

Yield: 12 muffins
Serving Size: 1 muffin
Exchanges:

		Nutrient Content per Serving			
		CAL	141	Na	215 (mg)
		PRO	4 (gm)	K	143 (mg)
Starch/Bread	1.5	Fat	3.8 (gm)	Fiber	2 (gm)
Fat	0.5	CHO	23 (gm)	Chol	1 (mg)

Ingredients

   1 CUP OAT BRAN, UNCOOKED
   1 CUP FLOUR
   ¼ CUP SUGAR
   1 TABLESPOON BAKING POWDER
   ½ TEASPOON BAKING SODA

½ TEASPOON CINNAMON
¼ TEASPOON SALT
½ CUP CURRANTS OR GOLDEN RAISINS
2 EGG WHITES
3 TABLESPOONS MARGARINE, MELTED
¼ CUP ORANGE JUICE
¾ CUP LOW-FAT BUTTERMILK
1 TEASPOON SHREDDED ORANGE PEEL

Method

1. Preheat oven to 375°F. Line 12 medium muffin cups with paper baking cups.
2. Combine oat bran, flour, sugar, baking powder, baking soda, cinnamon, and salt in medium bowl. Stir in currants.
3. Mix egg whites with a fork in a small bowl. Beat in margarine, orange juice, buttermilk, and orange peel. Add to dry ingredients; mix just until dry ingredients are moistened.
4. Fill muffin cups ¾ full. Bake 20–25 minutes or until light golden brown. Serve warm or cool completely, wrap, and freeze for later use.

Note: To make mini muffins, fill 24 small muffin cups and reduce baking time to 12–15 minutes. Low-fat buttermilk gives baked goods richness and tang that helps replace the traditionally high amount of fat. Skim milk may be substituted, but the texture and flavor of the baked good will be altered.

Herbed Biscuits

Yield: 12 biscuits
Serving Size: 1 biscuit

Exchanges:

Starch/Bread	1.0
Fat	1.0

Nutrient Content per Serving

CAL	125	Na	217 (mg)
PRO	3 (gm)	K	48 (mg)
Fat	4.2 (gm)	Fiber	0.8 (gm)
CHO	18 (gm)	Chol	1 (mg)

Ingredients

    2 CUPS ALL-PURPOSE FLOUR
    1 TABLESPOON BAKING POWDER
    ½ TEASPOON BAKING SODA
    ¼ TEASPOON SALT
    ¼ TEASPOON THYME LEAVES, CRUSHED
    ¼ TEASPOON ROSEMARY, CRUSHED
    ¼ TEASPOON BASIL LEAVES, CRUSHED
    ¼ CUP MARGARINE, CHILLED
    ¾ CUP LOW-FAT BUTTERMILK

Method

1. Heat oven to 400°F.
2. Combine flour, baking powder, baking soda, salt, thyme, rosemary, and basil in medium bowl.
3. Cut in margarine until size of coarse meal. Stir in buttermilk just until dry ingredients are moistened.
4. Knead dough on lightly floured surface 5 times. Roll out to ½-inch thickness. Cut with 2-inch round cutter or juice glass (but do not twist) to use all dough. Place 1 inch apart on ungreased cookie sheet. Bake 10–12 minutes or until golden brown. Serve warm.

Home-Style French Toast

Yield: 2 servings
Serving Size: ½ recipe
Exchanges:
Starch/Bread   1.5
Fat   1.0

Nutrient Content per Serving

CAL	174	Na	271 (mg)
PRO	6 (gm)	K	181 (mg)
Fat	6.6 (gm)	Fiber	1.5 (gm)
CHO	23 (gm)	*Chol	1 (mg)

*Add 137 mg if whole egg is used.

Ingredients

¼ CUP SKIM MILK
¼ CUP EGG SUBSTITUTE OR 1 EGG, BEATEN
⅛ TEASPOON NUTMEG, PREFERABLY FRESHLY GRATED
1 TABLESPOON MARGARINE
2 REGULAR OR 4 THIN SLICES WHOLE WHEAT BREAD
  (ABOUT 4 OUNCES)
1 TEASPOON POWDERED SUGAR
1 TEASPOON PRESERVES OR JAM

Method

1. Combine milk, egg substitute, and nutmeg in pie plate.
2. Heat margarine in nonstick skillet over medium heat. Dip bread in milk mixture on both sides, letting bread soak up all mixture.
3. Fry bread in margarine until golden brown on both sides, about 5 minutes. Sprinkle with sugar; serve with preserves.

Note: The family will love this French toast for Sunday morning breakfast.

Whole Grain Tofu Muffins

Yield: 1 dozen muffins
Serving Size: 1 muffin
Exchanges:
Starch/Bread   2.0
Fat   0.5

Nutrient Content per Serving

CAL	168	Na	169 (mg)
PRO	5 (gm)	K	86 (mg)
Fat	5.1 (gm)	Fiber	1.2 (gm)
CHO	27 (gm)	Chol	46 (mg)

Ingredients

8 OUNCES SOFT TOFU
2 EGGS
½ CUP HONEY
3 TABLESPOONS MARGARINE, MELTED
2 TEASPOONS CINNAMON
¼ TEASPOON SALT
1 CUP ALL-PURPOSE FLOUR
½ CUP ROLLED OATS, UNCOOKED
½ CUP WHOLE WHEAT FLOUR
1 TABLESPOON BAKING POWDER

Method

1. Heat oven to 425°F. Line 12 medium muffin tins with paper liners.
2. Combine tofu, eggs, honey, margarine, cinnamon, and salt in food processor fitted with steel blade or in bowl of electric mixer. Blend or heat until smooth.
3. Add remaining ingredients; process or beat just until dry ingredients are moistened.
4. Spoon into prepared muffin cups; bake 18–20 minutes or until golden brown and toothpick inserted in center comes out clean. Cool in pan 5 minutes; transfer to cooling rack. Serve warm or cool, or freeze for later use.

Meats: Beef, Pork, Veal, Lamb, Game

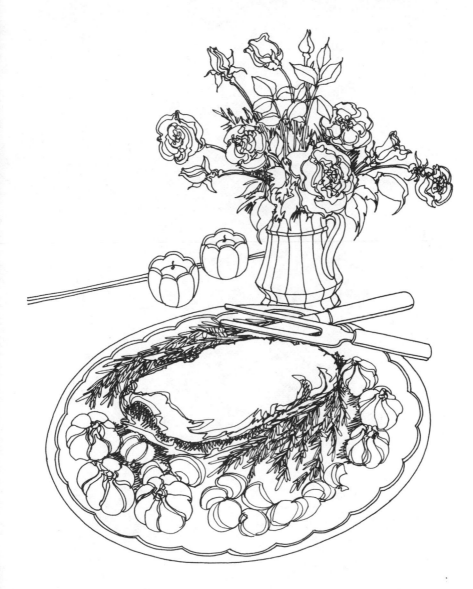

Veal Limone

		Nutrient Content per Serving			
Yield: 4 servings					
Serving Size: 3 ounces cooked veal		CAL	205	Na	92 (mg)
		PRO	29 (gm)	K	417 (mg)
Exchanges:		Fat	8.5 (gm)	Fiber	0 (gm)
Meat, lean	3.0	CHO	1 (gm)	Chol	84 (mg)
Fat	0.5				

Ingredients

1 POUND VEAL SCALLOPS, POUNDED TO ⅛-INCH
  THICKNESS
⅛ TEASPOON GROUND WHITE PEPPER
1 TABLESPOON SUNFLOWER MARGARINE
1 CLOVE GARLIC, MINCED
2 TABLESPOONS DRY WHITE WINE
2 TABLESPOONS LEMON JUICE
1 TABLESPOON CAPERS, RINSED AND DRAINED
1 TABLESPOON CHOPPED PARSLEY, PREFERABLY
  ITALIAN

Method

1. Season veal with pepper. Heat margarine in large nonstick skillet over medium-high heat.
2. Sauté veal (in batches if necessary so as not to crowd) until lightly browned, about 2 minutes per side. Remove to warm serving platter; cover with foil.
3. Add garlic to skillet; sauté 1 minute. Add wine, lemon juice, and capers to skillet. Increase heat to high and boil 1 minute. Pour over veal; sprinkle with parsley.

Pork in Apple-Brandy Glaze

Yield: 4 servings
Serving Size: 1 4-ounce pork patty
Exchanges:
Meat, lean   3.0

Nutrient Content per Serving

CAL	164	Na	194 (mg)
PRO	26 (gm)	K	484 (mg)
Fat	4.4 (gm)	Fiber	0 (gm)
CHO	4 (gm)	Chol	82 (mg)

Ingredients

    4 PORK TENDERLOIN PATTIES (ABOUT 4 OUNCES
      EACH)*
    ¼ TEASPOON SALT
    ⅛ TEASPOON GROUND WHITE PEPPER
    4 TEASPOONS APPLE CIDER JELLY
    2 TABLESPOONS BRANDY OR COGNAC
    1 TABLESPOON CHOPPED ITALIAN PARSLEY

Method

1. Sprinkle pork with salt and pepper. Spread evenly with apple jelly.
2. Heat large nonstick skillet over medium heat. Add pork and cook 5 minutes per side or until pork is cooked through. Remove to warm serving platter.
3. Add brandy to skillet; cook and stir until boiling and thickened. Pour over pork; sprinkle with parsley.

   *To make pork patties, cut on large tenderloin across grain into 4 4-ounce pieces and pound cut side down between pieces of wax paper to ½-inch thickness. (If tenderloin is in 2 smaller pieces, cut into 8 2-ounce pieces. Or ask butcher to prepare for you.)

Grilled Marinated Sirloin Steak

Yield: 4 servings	Nutrient Content per Serving			
Serving Size: 3 ounces cooked	CAL	182	Na	85 (mg)
steak	PRO	24 (gm)	K	400 (mg)
Exchanges:	Fat	8.1 (gm)	Fiber	0 (gm)
Meat, lean 3.0	CHO	1 (gm)	Chol	72 (mg)

Ingredients

    1 POUND BONELESS BEEF TOP SIRLOIN STEAK, CUT 1
      INCH THICK
    1 TABLESPOON BALSAMIC VINEGAR
    1 TABLESPOON TOMATO PASTE
    2 CLOVES GARLIC, MINCED
    1 TEASPOON EACH DRIED MARJORAM AND THYME
    ½ TEASPOON CRACKED BLACK PEPPERCORNS

Method

1. Place steak in shallow glass dish or pie plate.
2. Combine remaining ingredients; spread evenly over both sides
   of steak. Let stand at room temperature 30 minutes or cover
   and refrigerate up to 8 hours.
3. Grill or broil steak 4–5 inches from heat source 4 minutes per
   side for medium rare or to desired doneness.
4. Slice steak into thin strips; serve immediately.

Beef Sate with Peanut Dipping Sauce

Yield: 4 servings
Serving Size: ¼ recipe
Exchanges:
Meat, lean   3.0
Vegetable   1.0
Fat   1.0

Nutrient Content per Serving
CAL   237   Na   390 (mg)
PRO   24 (gm)   K   498 (mg)
Fat   12.5 (gm)   Fiber   1 (gm)
CHO   8 (gm)   Chol   58 (mg)

Ingredients

BAMBOO OR METAL SKEWERS
1 POUND BONELESS BEEF SIRLOIN STEAK, CUT 1 INCH
    THICK, WELL TRIMMED (ABOUT 12 OUNCES AFTER
    TRIMMING)
3 TABLESPOONS RICE WINE OR DRY SHERRY
2 TABLESPOONS REDUCED-SODIUM SOY SAUCE
1 TABLESPOON LIME JUICE
1 TABLESPOON GRATED ONION
1 TABLESPOON PEANUT OIL
1 TEASPOON SESAME OIL
1 TEASPOON SUGAR
2 LARGE CLOVES GARLIC, MINCED
½ TEASPOON RED PEPPER FLAKES
4 LARGE GREEN ONIONS WITH TOPS, CUT INTO 1-INCH
    LENGTHS
⅓ CUP EVAPORATED SKIM MILK
1 TABLESPOON CREAMY PEANUT BUTTER

Method

1. If using bamboo skewers, soak in cold water to cover while
   marinating meat. Cut meat into ⅛- to ¼-inch-wide strips;
   place in glass dish or plastic bag.
2. Combine wine, soy sauce, lime juice, onion, oils, sugar, garlic, and red pepper flakes; pour over meat. Cover dish or
   close bag securely and refrigerate 1–2 hours.

3. Drain marinade into small saucepan. Thread meat accordion-style onto skewers alternately with green onions. Grill over medium coals or broil 4–5 inches from heat source 6–8 minutes or until meat is no longer pink, turning once.
4. Meanwhile, add milk and peanut butter to reserved marinade. Simmer over low heat until thickened, stirring frequently. (Do not boil). Serve in small bowls for dipping.

Method-Microwave

1. Soak bamboo skewers in cold water to cover while marinating meat. Prepare meat and marinate as in steps 1 and 2 above.
2. Drain marinade into 2-cup glass measure. Thread meat accordion-style onto skewers alternately with green onions. Place across glass baking dish so that ends of skewers rest on edges of dish.
3. Add peanut butter and milk to marinade. Cook on high power 2–3 minutes or until thickened, stirring once. Let stand while cooking meat.
4. Cook meat on high power 4–5 minutes or until no longer pink, turning and rearranging skewers after 2 minutes. Serve with dipping sauce.

Note: Do not use skewers if preparing in the microwave oven. To further reduce sodium in the diet, look for low-salt peanut butters now available.

Steak au Poivre

Yield: 2 servings

Serving Size: 3 ounces cooked steak

Exchanges:

Meat, lean 3.0

Fat 0.5

Nutrient Content per Serving

CAL	199	Na	171 (mg)
PRO	25 (gm)	K	376 (mg)
Fat	10.4 (gm)	Fiber	0 (gm)
CHO	0 (gm)	Chol	72 (mg)

Ingredients

2 TENDERLOIN OR TOP SIRLOIN STEAKS, WELL TRIMMED (4 OUNCES EACH)
1 TEASPOON OLIVE OIL
¾ TEASPOON CRACKED BLACK PEPPERCORNS
¼ CUP DRY RED WINE
¼ CUP CANNED BEEF BROTH

Method

1. Brush steaks lightly on both sides with oil. Press peppercorns evenly onto both sides of steaks.
2. Heat nonstick skillet over medium-high heat until hot, about 3 minutes. Add steaks and quickly sear until medium rare, about 3 minutes per side for 1-inch steaks, 2 minutes for ¾-inch steaks.
3. Remove to warm plates; keep warm. Add wine and broth to skillet; cook until slightly reduced, about 2 minutes. Pour over steaks; serve immediately.

Note: This recipe is perfect for quick company fare for special guests.

Veal Marsala with Shiitake Mushrooms

Yield: 4 servings
Serving Size: ¼ recipe
Exchanges:
Meat, lean   4.0

Nutrient Content per Serving

CAL	212	Na	193 (mg)
PRO	29 (gm)	K	441 (mg)
Fat	9.2 (gm)	Fiber	0 (gm)
CHO	1 (gm)	Chol	84 (mg)

Ingredients

    1 POUND VEAL SCALLOPS, CUT ¼ INCH THICK
    ¼ TEASPOON SALT
    ¼ TEASPOON FRESHLY GROUND BLACK PEPPER
    3 TEASPOONS OLIVE OIL
    2 TABLESPOONS MINCED SHALLOT OR ONION
    3 OUNCES SHIITAKE OR BUTTON MUSHROOMS, STEMS
        DISCARDED, CAPS SLICED
    2 TABLESPOONS REDUCED-SODIUM CHICKEN BROTH
    2 TABLESPOONS MARSALA OR DRY RED WINE

Method

1. Sprinkle veal with salt and pepper.
2. Heat 2 teaspoons oil in large nonstick skillet over medium-high heat. Quickly sauté veal until lightly browned, about 2 minutes per side. Remove to warm serving plate; keep warm.
3. Add remaining 1 teaspoon oil to skillet. Sauté shallot and mushrooms, stirring often, until tender, about 4 minutes.
4. Add broth, marsala, and any juices that have accumulated from veal. Cook and stir until bubbly; pour over veal.

Hearty Yukon Stew

Yield: 6 cups (6 servings)
Serving Size: 1 cup
Exchanges:
Starch/Bread   2.0
Meat, lean   2.0
Vegetable   1.0

Nutrient Content per Serving

CAL	317	*Na	107 (mg)
PRO	32 (gm)	K	529 (mg)
Fat	6.1 (gm)	Fiber	3.7 (gm)
CHO	33 (gm)	Chol	95 (mg)

*Add 178 mg if optional salt is used.

Ingredients

1½ POUNDS BONELESS VENISON OR VEAL SHOULDER, CUT INTO 1½–INCH PIECES
3 TABLESPOONS FLOUR
½ TEASPOON SALT (OPTIONAL)
½ TEASPOON FRESHLY GROUND BLACK PEPPER
1 TABLESPOON OLIVE OIL
2 CLOVES GARLIC, MINCED
2 CUPS DRY RED WINE
1 CUP REDUCED-SODIUM CHICKEN BROTH OR WATER
1 TABLESPOON NO-SALT-ADDED TOMATO PASTE
2 CUPS (8 OUNCES) CARROTS, SLICED IN ½-INCH PIECES (4 MEDIUM CARROTS)
1 BAY LEAF
¾ POUND SMALL WHOLE WHITE ONIONS, PEELED (ABOUT 12)
8 OUNCES MEDIUM MUSHROOMS, STEMS TRIMMED
1 TABLESPOON CHOPPED FRESH THYME LEAVES OR 1 TEASPOON DRIED THYME
3 CUPS HOT COOKED YOLK-FREE EGG NOODLES, COOKED WITHOUT SALT OR FAT
CHOPPED PARSLEY (OPTIONAL)

Method

1. Dredge venison in flour combined with salt, if desired, and pepper. Heat oil in large nonstick skillet over medium-high heat. Brown venison in oil (in batches if necessary). Add garlic and cook for 1 minute.
2. Add wine, broth, and tomato paste; bring to a boil. Add carrots and bay leaf. Reduce heat; cover and simmer 30 minutes, stirring occasionally.
3. Add onions, mushrooms, and thyme; cover and simmer 30 minutes or until venison and onions are fork-tender. Simmer uncovered until sauce is desired consistency. Serve over noodles; sprinkle with parsley, if desired.

Method-Microwave

1. Dredge venison in flour combined with salt, if desired, and pepper. Place in 3-quart microwave-safe casserole dish. Stir in oil and garlic. Cover and cook on high power 5 minutes. Stir well; cover and continue to cook until no longer pink, about 4–5 minutes.
2. Add wine, broth, and tomato paste to dish. Stir in carrots and bay leaf. Cover and cook on high power 6–8 minutes. Reduce power to medium and continue to cook 28–30 minutes, stirring once.
3. Add onions, mushrooms, and thyme; cover and continue to cook on medium power 28–30 minutes or until venison and onions are fork-tender. Serve over noodles; sprinkle with parsley, if desired.

Note: Microwave version will have thinner consistency. If desired, strain off sauce into saucepan and cook over high heat until reduced. Stew may be covered tightly and refrigerated up to 5 days or frozen up to 4 months.

Roast Spring Lamb

Yield: About 2 pounds cooked lamb

Serving Size: 3 ounces cooked lamb

Exchanges:

Meat, lean   3.0

Nutrient Content per Serving

CAL	187	Na	64 (mg)
PRO	26 (gm)	K	308 (mg)
Fat	8.3 (gm)	Fiber	0 (gm)
CHO	0 (gm)	Chol	83 (mg)

Ingredients

  1 SIRLOIN HALF LEG OF LAMB, WELL-TRIMMED, BONED, AND BUTTERFLIED (TOP HALF OF LEG, 2½–3 POUNDS)
  3 CLOVES GARLIC, CUT INTO SLIVERS
  2 TEASPOONS ROSEMARY, CRUSHED
  1 TEASPOON CRACKED BLACK PEPPERCORNS

Method

1. Heat oven to 325°F.
2. Cut small, deep slits in lamb; insert 1 garlic silver in each slit. Rub surface of lamb with rosemary and pepper. Place on rack in shallow roasting pan. Roast until meat thermometer inserted in thickest part of meat registers 145°F (about 1 hour, depending on thickness of lamb). Let stand tented with foil 10 minutes before carving.
3. Thinly slice lamb across grain. Pour any accumulated juices from carving board over lamb slices. Serve immediately.

Note: The family will look forward to its Easter dinner when you make this recipe a tradition.

New Mexico–Style Flank Steak

Yield: 4 servings	Nutrient Content per Serving			
Serving Size: 3 ounces cooked	CAL	200	Na	70 (mg)
steak	PRO	21 (gm)	K	333 (mg)
Exchanges:	Fat	12.5 (gm)	Fiber	0 (gm)
Meat, medium-fat 3.0	CHO	0 (gm)	Chol	58 (mg)

Ingredients

   ¼ CUP TEQUILA
   2 TABLESPOONS LIME JUICE
   2 CLOVES GARLIC, MINCED
   ½ TEASPOON RED PEPPER SAUCE
   1 POUND FLANK STEAK
     FRESHLY GROUND BLACK PEPPER

Method

1. Combine tequila, lime juice, garlic, and red pepper sauce in shallow glass dish or heavy plastic bag.
2. Add steak; turn to coat. Marinate in refrigerator 6 hours or overnight.
3. Drain and discard marinade. Grill or broil steak 4–5 inches from heat source 4 minutes per side for medium rare or to desired doneness. Carve steak into thin slices across grain. Serve with pepper.

Pork Chops Paprikash

Yield: 4 servings	Nutrient Content per Serving			
Serving Size: ¼ recipe	CAL	230	Na	92 (mg)
Exchanges:	PRO	24 (gm)	K	407 (mg)
Meat, medium-fat 3.0	Fat	13.2 (gm)	Fiber	1.2 (gm)
Vegetable 1.0	CHO	4 (gm)	Chol	77 (mg)
Fat 1.0				

Ingredients

- 1 LARGE ONION, THINLY SLICED (8 OUNCES)
- 1 CLOVE GARLIC, MINCED
- 1 TEASPOON OLIVE OIL
- 4 CENTER CUT PORK CHOPS, CUT ½ INCH THICK, WELL TRIMMED (1¼ POUNDS)
- 2 TEASPOONS PAPRIKA, PREFERABLY SWEET
- ¼ TEASPOON HOT HUNGARIAN PAPRIKA OR CAYENNE PEPPER (OPTIONAL)
- ¼ CUP RINSED, DRAINED, AND SQUEEZED-DRY SAUERKRAUT (1½ OUNCES)

Method

1. Sauté onion and garlic in oil in nonstick skillet until very tender, about 6–8 minutes. Remove and reserve.
2. Sprinkle pork chops with sweet and hot paprika, if desired. Brown in same skillet over medium heat 3 minutes per side.
3. Combine onion mixture and sauerkraut; spoon evenly over chops. Sprinkle with additional paprika, if desired.
4. Cover and cook over low heat until pork chops are no longer pink, about 6–8 minutes.

Method-Microwave

1. Combine onion, garlic, and oil in shallow 2-quart baking dish. Cook uncovered on high power 4 minutes. Remove and reserve.

2. Sprinkle pork chops with sweet and hot paprika, if desired. Place in same baking dish with meaty portions toward outside of dish. Cover with wax paper. Cook on high power 5 minutes. Turn chops over. Combine onion mixture and sauerkraut; spoon over chops. Sprinkle with additional paprika, if desired. Cover with wax paper; cook on medium power until chops are no longer pink in center, 10–12 minutes.

Roast Brisket of Veal with Onion Sauce

Servings: Will vary depending on size of brisket. Each cooked pound of meat will yield about 5 servings.
Serving Size: 3 ounces cooked veal plus ¼ cup onion sauce

Nutrient Content per Serving

CAL	176	Na	103 (mg)
PRO	24 (gm)	K	460 (mg)
Fat	5.5 (gm)	Fiber	0.8 (gm)
CHO	6 (gm)	Chol	99 (mg)

Exchanges:
Meat, lean   3.0
Vegetable   1.0

Ingredients

1 VERY LARGE OR 2 MEDIUM ONIONS, SLICED (12 OUNCES)
1 VEAL BRISKET, WELL TRIMMED (ABOUT 3–3½ POUNDS)
½ TEASPOON FRESHLY GROUND BLACK PEPPER
1 CUP NO-SALT-ADDED CHILI SAUCE
1 BOTTLE OR CAN BEER (12 OUNCES)

(continued on page 182)

Method

1. Heat oven to 325°F.
2. Separate onion slices into rings. Scatter half over bottom of large roasting pan. Place brisket over onions; sprinkle with pepper. Sprinkle remaining onions over brisket. Stir chili sauce and beer together and pour over brisket.
3. Cover and bake until fork-tender, about 2½–3 hours, basting with pan juices 2 or 3 times.
4. Remove brisket to carving board. Skim fat from surface of pan juices. Transfer juices to saucepan and cook over high heat until slightly thickened and reduced to 2½ cups. Thinly slice brisket against the grain; pour ¼ cup onion sauce over each serving.

Note: Brisket is even better served the next day. Prepare on a weekend for a busy weeknight supper. Wrap brisket well in foil and chill before slicing. Chill sauce and remove fat when it has solidified. Reheat brisket and prepare sauce as directed in step 4 above.

Lamb over Minted Couscous

Yield: 2 servings
Serving Size: ½ recipe
Exchanges:

		Nutrient Content per Serving		
Starch/Bread	3.0	CAL	472	Na	152 (mg)
Meat, medium-fat	2.0	PRO	28 (gm)	K	1330 (mg)
Vegetable	1.0	Fat	20.1 (gm)	Fiber	6.1 (gm)
Fat	1.0	CHO	49 (gm)	Chol	77 (mg)

Ingredients

½ POUND GROUND LAMB
1 MEDIUM ONION, CHOPPED
1 CLOVE GARLIC, MINCED
1 TEASPOON CINNAMON
1 15-OUNCE CAN NO-SALT-ADDED TOMATO SAUCE
¼ CUP RAISINS OR CURRANTS
½ CUP REDUCED-SODIUM CHICKEN BROTH
⅓ CUP UNCOOKED COUSCOUS
2 TABLESPOONS CHOPPED FRESH MINT LEAVES OR 1
TEASPOON DRIED MINT
2 TABLESPOONS TOASTED SLIVERED ALMONDS

Method

1. Cook lamb, onion, and garlic in nonstick skillet until no longer pink. Drain well. Sprinkle with cinnamon.
2. Stir in tomato sauce and raisins; simmer uncovered 15 minutes, stirring occasionally.
3. While lamb is simmering, bring broth to a boil in small saucepan. Stir in couscous and mint; cover and let stand 5 minutes. Fluff with fork. Serve lamb over couscous; sprinkle with almonds.

Method-Microwave

1. Combine lamb, onion, and garlic in shallow 1½ quart-microwave-safe casserole dish. Cover with wax paper. Cook on high power until lamb is no longer pink, about 4–5 minutes, stirring once. Drain well. Sprinkle with cinnamon.
2. Add tomato sauce and raisins; cover with wax paper. Cook on high power 5 minutes; stir and reduce power to medium. Continue to cook 10 minutes, stirring once. Let stand, covered with wax paper, while preparing couscous.
3. Place broth in 1-cup glass measuring cup. Cook on high power until boiling, 1½–2 minutes. Stir in couscous and mint; cover with plastic wrap. Let stand 5 minutes or until liquid is absorbed. Fluff with fork. Serve lamb over couscous; sprinkle with almonds.

Minted Lamb Kabobs

Yield: 4 servings
Serving Size: 1 kabob
Exchanges:
Meat, lean   3.0

Nutrient Content per Serving

CAL	182	Na	68 (mg)
PRO	25 (gm)	K	315 (mg)
Fat	8 (gm)	Fiber	0 (gm)
CHO	1 (gm)	Chol	79 (mg)

Ingredients

> 1 POUND BONELESS LEG OF LAMB, CUT INTO 1-INCH CUBES
> ¾ CUP PLAIN LOW-FAT YOGURT
> 2 CLOVES GARLIC, MINCED
> 1 TABLESPOON CHOPPED FRESH MINT LEAVES OR 1 TEASPOON DRIED MINT
> ¼ TEASPOON POWDERED SAFFRON (OPTIONAL)
> ⅛ TEASPOON GROUND WHITE PEPPER

Method

1. Place lamb cubes in shallow glass dish or plastic bag. Combine remaining ingredients; mix well. Pour over lamb. Cover and refrigerate at least 2 hours or overnight.
2. Thread lamb onto skewers, reserving marinade. Broil or grill 6–8 inches from heat source, turning and basting with marinade several times.

Pacific Rim Omelet Rolls

		Nutrient Content per Serving		
Yield: 2 servings				
Serving Size: 1 omelet roll		CAL 231	Na	384 (mg)
Exchanges:		PRO 34 (gm)	K	968 (mg)
Meat, lean	4.0	Fat 7.4 (gm)	Fiber	2 (gm)
Vegetable	1.0	CHO 7 (gm)	Chol	219 (mg)

Ingredients

1 WHOLE EGG
1 EGG WHITE
2 TEASPOONS REDUCED-SODIUM SOY SAUCE, DIVIDED
NONSTICK VEGETABLE SPRAY
½ POUND LEAN GROUND PORK
1 LARGE CLOVE GARLIC, MINCED
½ TEASPOON RED PEPPER FLAKES
2 CUPS PACKED FRESH SPINACH LEAVES, SLICED
¼ CUP WATER
2 TEASPOONS CORNSTARCH

Method

1. Beat egg and egg white with 1 teaspoon of the soy sauce. Heat 8- or 9-inch nonstick skillet or crêpe pan over medium-high heat. Spray with vegetable spray. Pour in half of egg mixture, tilting skillet to form an even layer. Cook about 1 minute or until egg looks dry and bottom is golden brown. Slide out onto plate; repeat with remaining egg mixture.
2. Brown pork with garlic and red pepper in same skillet; pour off drippings. Add spinach; cook until wilted, 1–2 minutes.
3. Combine water, cornstarch, and remaining soy sauce; mix well. Pour into skillet, stirring until thickened. Spoon half of pork mixture down center of uncooked side of each omelet; roll up.

Marinated Skirt Steaks with Vegetable Chutney

Yield: 4 servings
Serving Size: ¼ recipe
Exchanges:

		Nutrient Content per Serving			
		CAL	272	Na	270 (mg)
		PRO	22 (gm)	K	453 (mg)
Meat, medium-fat	3.0	Fat	15 (gm)	Fiber	1.6 (gm)
Vegetable	1.0	CHO	13 (gm)	Chol	58 (mg)
Fruit	0.5				

Ingredients

- 1 POUND TRIMMED SKIRT OR FLANK STEAK
- 1 CAN OR BOTTLE BEER (12 OUNCES)
- 1 LARGE ONION, DICED ¼ INCH
- 2 TABLESPOONS CHOPPED PICKLED JALAPEÑO PEPPERS OR 1 LARGE FRESH JALAPEÑO PEPPER, CHOPPED
- 2 CLOVES GARLIC, MINCED
  FRESHLY GROUND BLACK PEPPER
- ¼ TEASPOON SALT
- 2 TEASPOONS OLIVE OIL
- ½ CUP DICED RED BELL PEPPER (¼ INCH)
- ½ CUP DICED YELLOW BELL PEPPER OR ADDITIONAL RED BELL PEPPER (¼ INCH)
- 2 TABLESPOONS ORANGE OR LIME MARMALADE
- 1 TEASPOON MINCED CRYSTALLIZED GINGER

Method

1. Place steak in shallow glass dish or heavy plastic bag. Add beer, onion, jalapeño pepper, and garlic. Turn steak in liquid. Cover dish or close bag securely and refrigerate at least 8 hours or up to 24 hours, turning several times.
2. Drain off liquid, reserving vegetables and meat separately. Sprinkle steak with salt and black pepper to taste.
3. Heat oil in small saucepan. Sauté drained vegetables in oil 3 minutes. Add remaining ingredients; cover and simmer 10

minutes. Uncover and continue to simmer until thickened, about 5 minutes. Cool to room temperature.
4. Grill or broil steak 5–6 inches from heat source to desired doneness, about 8 minutes for skirt steak and 10 minutes for flank steak for medium rare. Slice steak and serve with chutney.

Herb-Roasted Pork Tenderloin

Yield: 4 servings
Serving Size: ¼ recipe
Exchanges:
Meat, lean   3.0

Nutrient Content per Serving

CAL	151	Na	107 (mg)
PRO	26 (gm)	K	484 (mg)
Fat	4.6 (gm)	Fiber	0 (gm)
CHO	0 (gm)	Chol	82 (mg)

Ingredients

    1 POUND WHOLE PORK TENDERLOIN
    1 TABLESPOON COUNTRY-STYLE (GRAINY) DIJON
      MUSTARD
    1 TABLESPOON EACH CHOPPED FRESH MARJORAM
      OR OREGANO, THYME, SAGE, AND ROSEMARY
      LEAVES OR 1 TEASPOON EACH DRIED
    ½ TEASPOON FRESHLY GROUND BLACK PEPPER

Method

1. Heat oven to 450°F.
2. Spread tenderloin with mustard. Combine herbs; pat evenly onto tenderloin. Sprinkle with pepper.
3. Place on rack in shallow roasting pan. Place in oven and immediately reduce oven temperature to 350°F. Roast until meat thermometer inserted in thickest part of tenderloin registers 145°F, about 30–40 minutes, depending on size of tenderloin. Let stand on carving board 5 minutes. Slice and serve immediately.

Alaskan-Style Rabbit Ragout

Yield: 4 servings
Serving Size: ¼ recipe
Exchanges:

Starch/Bread	0.5
Meat, lean	4.0
Vegetable	1.0

Nutrient Content per Serving

CAL	283	*Na	56 (mg)
PRO	32 (gm)	K	463 (mg)
Fat	12.1 (gm)	Fiber	2.7 (gm)
CHO	11 (gm)	Chol	83 (mg)

*Add 267 mg if optional salt is used.

Ingredients

  1 RABBIT, ABOUT 2½ POUNDS, CUT UP (DOMESTIC
    RATHER THAN WILD RABBIT)
  3 TABLESPOONS ALL-PURPOSE FLOUR
  ½ TEASPOON SALT (OPTIONAL)
  ¼ TEASPOON FRESHLY GROUND BLACK PEPPER
  1 TABLESPOON OLIVE OIL
  1 LARGE ONION, CUT INTO ½-INCH WEDGES
  2 CLOVES GARLIC, MINCED
  1 CUP DRY WHITE WINE
  1 CUP REDUCED-SODIUM CHICKEN BROTH OR
    HOMEMADE (PAGE 118)
  6 OUNCES SMALL FRESH MUSHROOMS, STEMS
    TRIMMED
  1 BAY LEAF
  1 TEASPOON DRIED THYME LEAVES, CRUSHED

Method

1. Dredge rabbit pieces in flour combined with salt, if desired, and pepper.
2. Heat oil in large nonstick skillet. Brown rabbit on all sides, about 10 minutes. Remove rabbit; add onion and garlic to skillet. Sauté until tender, about 4 minutes. Add remaining ingredients; bring to a boil.
3. Return rabbit to skillet; reduce heat, cover, and simmer until rabbit is tender, 50–60 minutes, stirring occasionally.

Method-Microwave

1. Prepare rabbit as directed in step 1 above.
2. Place in 13-by-9-inch glass baking dish; add onion and garlic. Drizzle with oil. Cover with wax paper; cook on high power 5 minutes. Add remaining ingredients; cover with vented plastic wrap.
3. Cook on high power 20–22 minutes or until rabbit is tender, rotating dish once after 12 minutes. Let stand covered, 5 minutes.

Poultry

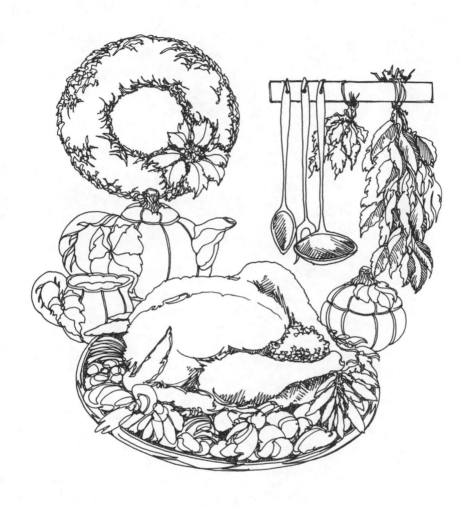

Stuffed Grilled Turkey Tenderloin

Yield: 4 servings
Serving Size: ½ tenderloin
Exchanges:
Meat, lean   3.0

Nutrient Content per Serving

CAL	148	Na	177 (mg)
PRO	28 (gm)	K	358 (mg)
Fat	1.9 (gm)	Fiber	1 (gm)
CHO	4 (gm)	Chol	77 (mg)

Ingredients

2 SMALL TURKEY TENDERLOINS, ABOUT ½ POUND
   EACH
   NONSTICK VEGETABLE SPRAY
1 CUP CHOPPED ONION
2 CLOVES GARLIC, MINCED
1 4-OUNCE CAN CHOPPED GREEN CHILES OR
   JALAPEÑO PEPPERS, AS DESIRED (¼ CUP)
½ CUP COARSELY CHOPPED CILANTRO
1 TEASPOON OLIVE OIL

Method

1. Cut deep pocket horizontally in side of each tenderloin, making sure not to cut all the way through.
2. Spray nonstick skillet with vegetable spray. Sauté onion and garlic until softened, about 3 minutes. Stir in green chiles and cilantro.
3. Stuff onion mixture into pockets in tenderloins; secure with metal skewer or wooden picks. Brush tenderloins lightly with oil.
4. Grill, covered, over medium coals or broil 6 inches from heat source 15 minutes per side or until tenderloins are cooked through. Cut into ½-inch slices.

Timely Turkey Tostados

Yield: 4 tostados
Serving Size: 1 tostado
Exchanges:

Starch/Bread	1.0
Meat, medium-fat	1.0
Vegetable	1.0
Fat	0.5

Nutrient Content per Serving

CAL	210	Na	359 (mg)
PRO	12 (gm)	K	214 (mg)
Fat	8.8 (gm)	Fiber	2 (gm)
CHO	21 (gm)	Chol	28 (mg)

Ingredients

½ POUND GROUND TURKEY
½ CUP COARSELY CHOPPED ONION
1 CLOVE GARLIC, MINCED
¼ CUP SALSA OR PICANTE SAUCE
¼ CUP REDUCED-SODIUM CHICKEN BROTH
1 TEASPOON CHILI POWDER
½ TEASPOON CUMIN SEEDS OR ¼ TEASPOON GROUND
  CUMIN
4 6-INCH FLOUR TORTILLAS
2 TABLESPOONS COARSELY CHOPPED CILANTRO
¼ CUP (1 OUNCE) SHREDDED REDUCED-FAT CHEDDAR
  OR MONTEREY JACK CHEESE
½ CUP SHREDDED LETTUCE
¼ CUP CHOPPED TOMATO
  CHOPPED FRESH JALAPEÑO PEPPERS (OPTIONAL)

Method

1. Cook turkey, onion, and garlic in 10-inch skillet over medium heat until no longer pink. Drain.
2. Add salsa, broth, chili powder, and cumin seeds. Simmer uncovered until most of liquid is evaporated, about 10–12 minutes, stirring occasionally.
3. While turkey mixture simmers, broil tortillas about 4–5 inches from heat source, until very crisp and golden brown, turning occasionally.

4. Stir cilantro into turkey mixture. Top each tortilla with ¼ cup turkey mixture, 1 tablespoon cheese, 2 tablespoons lettuce, and 1 tablespoon tomato. Sprinkle with peppers, if desired.

Method-Microwave

1. Crumble turkey into shallow 2-quart microwave-safe baking dish. Stir in onion and garlic. Cook uncovered on high power 3–4 minutes or until no longer pink, stirring once. Drain.
2. Add salsa, broth, chili powder, and cumin seeds. Cook on high power uncovered 6–8 minutes or until most of liquid is absorbed, stirring once.
3. Prepare tortillas and assemble tostados as in steps 3 and 4 above.

Note: Keep salsa on hand as a condiment for adding zip to many recipes. Avoid the prepared taco seasoning mixes, which are high in sodium.

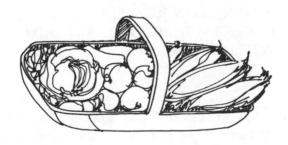

Heartland Stuffed Peppers

Yield: 4 servings
Serving Size: 1 stuffed pepper
Exchanges:
Starch/Bread 1.0
Meat, lean 4.0
Vegetable 2.0

Nutrient Content per Serving

CAL	345	*Na	200 (mg)
PRO	36 (gm)	K	618 (mg)
Fat	9.5 (gm)	Fiber	6 (gm)
CHO	30 (gm)	Chol	82 (mg)

*Add 267 mg if optional salt is used.

Ingredients

4 LARGE BELL PEPPERS, ANY COMBINATION OF RED,
   YELLOW, OR GREEN (ABOUT 1½ POUNDS)
¾ POUND GROUND RAW TURKEY
1 CUP CHOPPED ONION
1 GARLIC CLOVE, MINCED
1½ TEASPOONS PAPRIKA
1½ TEASPOONS DRIED SAGE
½ TEASPOON SALT (OPTIONAL)
½ TEASPOON HOT PEPPER SAUCE
1 CUP COOKED BROWN RICE
1 CUP FROZEN CORN KERNELS
½ CUP (4 OUNCES) SHREDDED PART-SKIM
   MOZZARELLA CHEESE

Method

1. Preheat oven to 350°F. Cut tops off peppers ½ inch from stem end. Discard membranes and seeds. Chop tops; discard stems.
2. Parboil pepper bottoms in boiling water 4 minutes. Drain well and stand upright in shallow baking dish.
3. Cook turkey with onion and garlic in skillet until no longer pink. Add paprika, sage, salt, pepper sauce, and chopped pepper tops. Cook 1 minute.
4. Stir in rice, frozen corn, and cheese. Pack into pepper cups. Bake uncovered 30 minutes or until heated through.

Method-Microwave

1. Prepare peppers as directed in step 1. Place in 8-inch square glass baking dish. Cover with plastic wrap.
2. Cook on high power 4–5 minutes. Remove and let stand.
3. Crumble turkey into shallow 2-quart microwave-safe dish. Stir in onion and garlic. Cover with vented plastic wrap; cook on high power 3 minutes. Stir; continue to cook 2 minutes. Drain. Add paprika, sage, salt, pepper sauce, chopped pepper tops, rice, frozen corn, and cheese.
4. Pack into pepper cups; cover with vented plastic wrap. Cook on high power 12–15 minutes, rotating dish once. Let stand loosely covered 5 minutes.

Sauté of Chicken with Caramelized Onions

Yield: 4 servings
Serving Size: ½ chicken breast
Exchanges:
Meat, lean 3.0
Vegetable 1.0

Nutrient Content per Serving

CAL	163	Na	96 (mg)
PRO	26 (gm)	K	307 (mg)
Fat	4.2 (gm)	Fiber	1 (gm)
CHO	4 (gm)	Chol	68 (mg)

Ingredients

    1 TEASPOON OLIVE OIL
    2 LARGE ONIONS, THINLY SLICED, SEPARATED INTO RINGS (12 OUNCES)
    2 WHOLE CHICKEN BREASTS, SPLIT, BONED, AND SKINNED (1 POUND)
    2 TEASPOONS COUNTRY-STYLE DIJON MUSTARD
    1 TEASPOON CRACKED BLACK PEPPERCORNS

(continued on page 198)

Method

1. Heat oil in large nonstick skillet.
2. Sauté onions over medium-low heat until tender and golden, about 15 minutes, stirring occasionally. Remove from skillet with slotted spatula; reserve.
3. Spread chicken evenly with mustard; sprinkle with pepper. Sauté in same skillet over medium heat 5 minutes per side, or until cooked through.
4. Pour reserved onions over chicken; heat through. Serve with additional cracked pepper, if desired.

Method-Microwave

1. Toss onions with oil in 2-quart microwave-safe dish. Cover with vented plastic wrap.
2. Cook on high power 7–9 minutes, stirring once. Remove from dish with slotted spatula; reserve.
3. Spread chicken evenly with mustard; sprinkle with pepper. Place in same dish with meaty portions toward outer edges. Cover with vented plastic wrap. Cook on high power 7–9 minutes, rotating dish once.
4. Return onions to dish; cook at high power uncovered 1 minute. Serve with additional pepper, if desired.

Note: This dish is particularly good in late spring when sweet onions such as Vidalia, Walla Walla, and Texas 1015 are in season.

Grilled Orange-Mustard Chicken

Yield: 2 servings
Serving Size: ½ chicken breast
Exchanges:
Meat, lean   3.0
Fruit   1.0

Nutrient Content per Serving

CAL	193	Na	128 (mg)
PRO	27 (gm)	K	296 (mg)
Fat	3.3 (gm)	Fiber	0 (gm)
CHO	12 (gm)	Chol	72 (mg)

Ingredients

1 WHOLE CHICKEN BREAST, SPLIT, BONED, AND
SKINNED
¼ CUP ORANGE JUICE
2 TABLESPOONS ORANGE-FLAVORED LIQUEUR
2 TEASPOONS COUNTRY-STYLE DIJON MUSTARD
1 TABLESPOON CHOPPED FRESH THYME LEAVES OR
1 TEASPOON DRIED THYME
1 CLOVE GARLIC, MINCED
ORANGE WEDGES

Method

1. Place chicken in shallow glass dish or plastic bag.
2. Combine remaining ingredients; pour over chicken.
3. Cover and refrigerate 1–2 hours. Drain chicken, reserving marinade.
4. Grill covered over medium coals or broil 4–5 inches from heat source 5 minutes per side or until chicken is cooked through, basting occasionally with marinade. Garnish with orange wedges.

Note: Liqueurs can add lots of flavor to recipes without adding any fat. The raw alcohol flavor will burn off during cooking.

Basque-Style Chicken

Yield: 4 servings
Serving Size: ½ chicken breast
Exchanges:
Meat, lean 3.0
Vegetable 1.0

Nutrient Content per Serving

CAL	191	*Na	67 (mg)
PRO	27 (gm)	K	293 (mg)
Fat	5.4 (gm)	Fiber	1 (gm)
CHO	7 (gm)	Chol	72 (mg)

*Add 133 mg if optional salt is used.

Ingredients

2 WHOLE CHICKEN BREASTS, SKINNED AND SPLIT (BONE IN) (1¼ POUNDS)
2 TABLESPOONS FLOUR
1 TEASPOON PAPRIKA
1 TEASPOON THYME
½ TEASPOON FRESHLY GROUND BLACK PEPPER
¼ TEASPOON SALT (OPTIONAL)
2 TEASPOONS OLIVE OIL
1 LARGE ONION, COARSELY CHOPPED (ABOUT 8 OUNCES)
2 CLOVES GARLIC, MINCED
1 CUP DRY WHITE WINE
1 BAY LEAF
1 TABLESPOON FINELY CHOPPED DRAINED ROASTED RED PEPPER OR PIMIENTO
2 TABLESPOONS CHOPPED PARSLEY

Method

1. Dredge chicken in flour combined with paprika, thyme, pepper, and salt, if desired.
2. Heat oil in large nonstick skillet with cover. Brown chicken over medium heat, about 4 minutes per side. Remove chicken and reserve.
3. Sauté onion and garlic in skillet until tender, about 3 minutes. Add wine; bring to a boil, stirring constantly.

4. Return chicken to skillet; add bay leaf. Cover and simmer over low heat until cooked through, about 20 minutes. Discard bay leaf. Sprinkle with parsley. Serve with rice or pasta, if desired.

Method-Microwave

1. Sprinkle chicken with paprika, thyme, pepper, and salt, if desired.
2. Toss onion and garlic with oil in shallow 2-quart microwave-safe dish. Cover and cook on high power 3 minutes. Stir flour into onion mixture.
3. Arrange chicken over onion mixture, meaty portions toward outer edges of dish. Add bay leaf. Pour wine over chicken. Cover and cook on high power 9 minutes.
4. Turn chicken over; cover and cook on high power 6–8 minutes or until chicken is cooked through. Discard bay leaf. Sprinkle with parsley. Serve with rice or pasta, if desired.

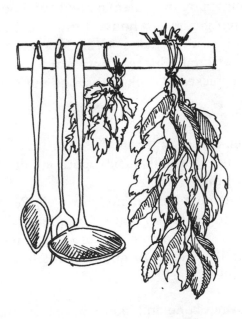

Teriyaki Chicken Breast

Yield: 4 servings
Serving size: ½ chicken breast
Exchanges:
Meat, lean   3.0

Nutrient Content per Serving

CAL	136	Na	210 (mg)
PRO	25 (gm)	K	215 (mg)
Fat	2.8 (gm)	Fiber	0 (gm)
CHO	0 (gm)	Chol	68 (mg)

Ingredients

   2 WHOLE CHICKEN BREASTS, SPLIT, BONED, AND
     SKINNED (1 POUND)
   ⅓ CUP DRY SHERRY
   2 TABLESPOONS REDUCED-SODIUM SOY SAUCE
   1 LARGE GARLIC CLOVE, MINCED
   ¼ TEASPOON RED PEPPER FLAKES

Method

1. Place chicken breasts in shallow glass dish.
2. Combine remaining ingredients; mix well. Pour over chicken. Cover and refrigerate 2–8 hours, turning chicken over once.
3. Drain and discard marinade. Grill chicken covered over medium coals, or broil 6 inches from heat source 5 minutes per side or until chicken is cooked through but still tender.

Method-Microwave

1. Place chicken breasts in shallow 2-quart microwave-safe dish or 10-inch pie plate with meaty portions of chicken toward outer edge of dish.
2. Combine remaining ingredients; mix well. Pour over chicken. Cover and refrigerate 2–8 hours, turning chicken over once.
3. Drain and discard marinade. Cover with vented plastic wrap. Cook on high power 8–10 minutes, rotating dish once. Let stand 3 minutes.

Note: Learn how to bone and skin chicken breasts to save food dollars. Whole chickens are still the most economical, but bone-in chicken breasts are often on sale.

Chicken Vesuvio

Yield: 4 servings
Serving Size: ¼ chicken with
3 ounces potato
Exchanges:
Starch/Bread   1.0
Meat, lean   4.0

Nutrient Content per Serving

CAL	297	Na	104 (mg)
PRO	34 (gm)	K	509 (mg)
Fat	10.7 (gm)	Fiber	1 (gm)
CHO	14 (gm)	Chol	100 (mg)

Ingredients

1 BROILER-FRYER CHICKEN, QUARTERED AND
SKINNED (ABOUT 3 POUNDS)
2 TEASPOONS EXTRA-VIRGIN OLIVE OIL
1 TABLESPOON CHOPPED FRESH ROSEMARY OR 1
TEASPOON DRIED ROSEMARY
3 LARGE CLOVES GARLIC, MINCED
¼ TEASPOON FRESHLY GROUND BLACK PEPPER
1 LARGE BAKING POTATO, PEELED AND CUT INTO
2-INCH PIECES (12 OUNCES)
3 TABLESPOONS CHOPPED ITALIAN PARSLEY
½ TEASPOON SHREDDED LEMON PEEL

Method

1. Preheat oven to 375°F. Brush chicken with oil; sprinkle with
   rosemary, 2 cloves garlic, and pepper.
2. Place in ovenproof casserole dish or small roasting pan. Place
   potato pieces around chicken. Cover with foil. Bake 30 minutes.
3. Uncover; baste with pan juices and continue to bake 20 minutes or until chicken and potatoes are tender.
4. Combine parsley, lemon peel, and remaining clove garlic;
   sprinkle over chicken.

Note: There is so much good garlic flavor in this recipe that the
salt is not missed. The traditional Italian gremolata garnish of
parsley, lemon peel, and raw garlic gives a burst of fresh flavor
and texture.

West Coast Chicken Breast

Yield: 4 servings
Serving Size: 1 stuffed chicken breast
Exchanges:
Meat, lean   3.0

Nutrient Content per Serving

CAL	171	Na	112 (mg)
PRO	26 (gm)	K	235 (mg)
Fat	5.8 (gm)	Fiber	0.5 (gm)
CHO	2 (gm)	Chol	68 (mg)

Ingredients

   2 WHOLE CHICKEN BREASTS, SPLIT, BONED, AND
      SKINNED (1 POUND)
   ¼ CUP CHOPPED SUN-DRIED TOMATOES IN OIL, OR
      WELL-DRAINED OR SLICED ROASTED RED PEPPERS
   ¼ CUP BASIL LEAVES, THINLY SLICED
   1 GARLIC CLOVE, MINCED
   1 TABLESPOON MARGARINE, MELTED
   ¼ TEASPOON FRESHLY GROUND BLACK PEPPER
   ¼ TEASPOON PAPRIKA
   ¼ CUP FRESH WHOLE WHEAT BREAD CRUMBS

Method

1. Preheat oven to 450°F.
2. Pound chicken to ¼-inch thickness. Combine tomatoes, basil, and garlic. Spread evenly over chicken breasts; roll up and place seam side down in shallow baking dish.
3. Combine margarine, pepper, and paprika. Brush evenly over chicken rolls. Sprinkle with bread crumbs.
4. Bake 15–18 minutes or until chicken is tender and crumbs are browned.

Note: This chicken is elegant enough to serve at a special dinner party. Prepare chicken and place on baking sheet; refrigerate loosely covered up to 4 hours before baking. Add 2 minutes to baking time for chilled chicken breasts.

Game Hens with Chutney-Mustard Glaze

Yield: 2 servings
Serving Size: ½ hen
Exchanges:
Meat, lean   4.0
Fruit   1.0

Nutrient Content per Serving

CAL	288	Na	209 (mg)
PRO	37 (gm)	K	360 (mg)
Fat	9.6 (gm)	Fiber	0 (gm)
CHO	11 (gm)	Chol	113 (mg)

Ingredients

1 CORNISH GAME HEN, SPLIT AND SKINNED (ABOUT 1¼ POUNDS)
2 TABLESPOONS CHOPPED MANGO CHUTNEY
2 TEASPOONS COUNTRY-STYLE DIJON MUSTARD

Method

1. Heat oven to 325°F.
2. Place hen halves meaty side up on rack in shallow roasting pan. Combine chutney and mustard; brush about ⅓ of mixture over hen.
3. Bake 50–60 minutes or until hen is tender, brushing twice more with chutney mixture.

Method-Microwave

1. Place hen halves meaty side up in shallow microwave-safe dish. Combine chutney and mustard; brush ⅔ of mixture over hen.
2. Cover with wax paper; cook on high power until hen is tender, 8–10 minutes, rotating dish once. Brush with remaining chutney mixture. Let stand, covered with wax paper, 5 minutes.

Coq au Vin

Yield: 4 servings	Nutrient Content per Serving
Serving Size: ¼ recipe	CAL 306 *Na 119 (mg)
Exchanges:	PRO 35 (gm) K 448 (mg)
Meat, lean 4.0	Fat 12.5 (gm) Fiber 2.7 (gm)
Vegetable 2.0	CHO 12 (gm) Chol 100 (mg)

*Add 133 mg if optional salt is used.

Ingredients

1 BROILER-FRYER CHICKEN, CUT INTO QUARTERS
AND SKINNED (ABOUT 3 POUNDS)
3 TABLESPOONS FLOUR
¼ TEASPOON SALT (OPTIONAL)
¼ TEASPOON FRESHLY GROUND BLACK PEPPER
1 TABLESPOON OLIVE OIL
8 SMALL WHITE BOILING ONIONS, PEELED (1-INCH
DIAMETER, 8 OUNCES)
1 TEASPOON SUGAR
2 CLOVES GARLIC, MINCED
8 OUNCES MEDIUM TO SMALL MUSHROOMS, STEMS
TRIMMED
1 CUP DRY RED WINE
1 CUP REDUCED-SODIUM CHICKEN BROTH
1 BAY LEAF
1 TEASPOON DRIED THYME
CHOPPED ITALIAN OR REGULAR PARSLEY

Method

1. Dredge chicken pieces in flour combined with salt, if desired,
   and pepper, using all of mixture. Heat oil in large nonstick
   skillet over medium heat. Brown chicken in oil, about 3 minutes per side.
2. Remove chicken; reserve. Add onions to drippings; sprinkle
   with sugar. Sauté until lightly browned. Add garlic and mushrooms; sauté 2 minutes.

3. Add wine, broth, bay leaf, and thyme; bring to a boil. Add chicken; reduce heat, cover, and simmer 40 minutes or until chicken is tender.
4. Transfer chicken and vegetables to 4 shallow bowls. Reduce sauce over high heat to desired consistency. Discard bay leaf; pour sauce over chicken. Sprinkle with parsley.

Note: This is a lightened version of the French classic that will perfume the whole house with a rustic aroma.

Spicy Chicken Thighs

		Nutrient Content per Serving			
Yield: 4 servings					
Serving Size: ¼ recipe		CAL	209	Na	167 (mg)
Exchanges:		PRO	25 (gm)	K	326 (mg)
Meat, lean	3.0	Fat	9.3 (gm)	Fiber	0.1 (gm)
Milk, skim	0.5	CHO	5 (gm)	Chol	81 (mg)

Ingredients

  1½ POUNDS CHICKEN THIGHS, SKINNED (4 LARGE OR 8 SMALL)
  1 8-OUNCE CONTAINER PLAIN LOW-FAT YOGURT
  ¼ CUP HOT SALSA, PICANTE SAUCE, OR JALAPEÑO RELISH
  1 TABLESPOON CURRY POWDER
  1 TEASPOON GROUND CUMIN

Method

1. Place chicken in glass dish. Combine yogurt, salsa, curry powder, and cumin. Pour over chicken, turning to coat. Cover and refrigerate at least 6 hours or overnight.
2. Heat oven to 375°F. Bake chicken and sauce uncovered 40–45 minutes, or until tender and no longer pink.

(continued on page 208)

Method-Microwave

1. Prepare and marinate chicken as in step 1 above, placing meaty portions of chicken toward outer edges of dish.
2. Cover dish with waxed paper. Cook on high power 10–12 minutes or until chicken is tender and no longer pink, rotating dish once.

Note: The heat of the salsa (hot, medium, or mild) will dictate the spice level in this recipe. Use what your family prefers. Some salsas will become hotter the longer they are kept in the refrigerator, so beware.

Ragout of Chicken, Sweet Potato, and Broccoli

Yield: 4 servings
Serving size: ¼ recipe
Exchanges:
Starch/Bread   2.0
Meat, lean   3.0
Fat   0.5

Nutrient Content per Serving

CAL	338	*Na	98 (mg)
PRO	26 (gm)	K	541 (mg)
Fat	12.6 (gm)	Fiber	3.9 (gm)
CHO	30 (gm)	Chol	78 (mg)

*Add 133 mg if optional salt is used.

Ingredients

1½ POUNDS CHICKEN THIGHS, SKINNED (4 LARGE OR 8 SMALL)
2 TABLESPOONS FLOUR
1 TEASPOON PAPRIKA, PREFERABLY HUNGARIAN
¼ TEASPOON FRESHLY GROUND BLACK PEPPER
¼ TEASPOON SALT (OPTIONAL)
1 TABLESPOON OLIVE OIL
1 LARGE ONION, HALVED LENGTHWISE AND SLICED CROSSWISE (6 OUNCES)

2 CLOVES GARLIC, MINCED
1 10½-OUNCE CAN REDUCED-SODIUM CHICKEN
BROTH OR 1⅓ CUPS HOMEMADE (PAGE 118)
1 BAY LEAF
2 MEDIUM SWEET POTATOES, PEELED AND
QUARTERED (1 POUND)
3 CUPS BROCCOLI FLORETS (6 OUNCES)
1 TEASPOON FINELY GRATED LEMON PEEL
(OPTIONAL)

Method

1. Dredge chicken in flour combined with paprika, pepper, and salt, if desired, patting in flour to use all.
2. Heat oil in large, deep skillet over medium heat. Sauté chicken in oil until lightly browned, about 3–4 minutes per side. Add onion and garlic; cook 1 minute.
3. Add broth, bay leaf, and potatoes. Cover and simmer over low heat 30 minutes. Tuck in broccoli, cover, and continue to simmer until chicken and potatoes are tender and broccoli is crisp-tender, about 8 minutes. Remove chicken and vegetables to serving platter; boil pan juices over high heat until thickened, about 5 minutes. Spoon over chicken and vegetables; sprinkle with lemon peel, if desired.

Method-Microwave

1. Prepare chicken as in step 1 above.
2. Place chicken in 3-quart microwave-safe casserole dish. Drizzle with oil. Cover and cook on high power 5 minutes. Add onion and garlic; cover and cook 2 minutes.
3. Add broth, bay leaf, and potatoes. Cover and cook on high power 5 minutes. Reduce power to medium and cook 25 minutes. Tuck in broccoli; cover and continue cooking on medium until chicken and potatoes are tender and broccoli is crisp-tender, 5–7 minutes. Remove chicken and vegetables to serving platter; reduce juices on stove in saucepan to desired consistency. Spoon over chicken and vegetables; sprinkle with lemon peel, if desired.

Chicken in Mole Sauce

Yield: 6 servings

Serving Size: ⅙ recipe

Exchanges:

Starch/Bread   2.0

Meat, Lean   3.0

Nutrient Content per Serving

CAL	313	Na	164 (mg)
PRO	32 (gm)	K	603 (mg)
Fat	5.1 (gm)	Fiber	2.5 (gm)
CHO	34 (gm)	Chol	76 (mg)

Ingredients

    1 LARGE ONION, COARSELY CHOPPED (8 OUNCES)
    2 CLOVES GARLIC, MINCED
    2 TEASPOONS OLIVE OR VEGETABLE OIL
    1 15-OUNCE CAN NO-SALT-ADDED TOMATO SAUCE
   ⅓ CUP PREPARED SALSA, PICANTE SAUCE, OR
      JALAPEÑO RELISH
    4 TEASPOONS UNSWEETENED COCOA
    1 TEASPOON GROUND CUMIN
     DASH OF ALLSPICE
2½ POUNDS CHICKEN BREAST HALVES AND/OR
      CHICKEN THIGHS, SKINNED
   ⅓ CUP COARSELY CHOPPED CILANTRO
    3 CUPS COOKED WHITE RICE (COOKED WITHOUT
      SALT OR FAT)

Method

1. Sauté onion and garlic in oil in large nonstick skillet until tender, about 4 minutes. Add tomato sauce, salsa, cocoa, cumin, and allspice. Bring to a boil, stirring well.
2. Add chicken; reduce heat. Cover and simmer until chicken is tender, about 25 minutes. Remove chicken to serving platter with rice. Stir sauce; pour over chicken and rice. Sprinkle with cilantro.

Method-Microwave

1. Toss onion and garlic with oil in 2½-quart microwave-safe casserole dish. Cover and cook on high power 3 minutes. Stir in tomato sauce, salsa, cocoa, cumin, and allspice. Cover and cook on high power 4 minutes.
2. Add chicken; spoon sauce over. Cover and cook on high power 20–24 minutes, or until chicken is tender, rearranging chicken with meaty parts toward edges of casserole halfway through cooking. Remove chicken to serving platter with rice. Spoon sauce over chicken and rice. Sprinkle with cilantro.

Note: Jalapeño relish varies from hot to super hot. If using this product for the first time, cut down on the amount, and taste and adjust as necessary.

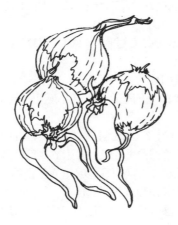

Georgian-Style Country Captain Chicken

Yield: 4 servings
Serving Size: ¼ recipe
Exchanges:
Meat, lean 4.0
Vegetable 2.0
Fruit 0.5
**Fat

Nutrient Content per Serving

CAL	306	*Na	117 (mg)
PRO	34 (gm)	K	588 (mg)
Fat	12.0 (gm)	Fiber	1.3 (gm)
CHO	15 (gm)	Chol	100 (mg)

*Add 267 mg if optional salt is used.
**Add 0.5 if optional almonds are used.

Ingredients

1 BROILER-FRYER CHICKEN (3 POUNDS), SKINNED AND CUT INTO 8 PIECES
2 TEASPOONS CURRY POWDER
½ TEASPOON SALT (OPTIONAL)
½ TEASPOON GROUND RED PEPPER (CAYENNE)
1 TABLESPOON OLIVE OIL
1 MEDIUM ONION, CUT INTO THIN WEDGES (6 OUNCES)
2 CLOVES GARLIC, MINCED
1 LARGE GREEN PEPPER (6 OUNCES), CUT INTO 1-INCH PIECES
1 15-OUNCE CAN NO-SALT-ADDED TOMATOES, UNDRAINED AND COARSELY CHOPPED
¼ CUP DRIED CURRANTS OR RAISINS
½ TEASPOON DRIED THYME
2 TABLESPOONS TOASTED SLICED ALMONDS (OPTIONAL)

Method

1. Sprinkle chicken pieces with curry powder, salt, if desired, and red pepper.
2. Heat oil in large nonstick skillet. Brown chicken in oil on all sides, about 10 minutes. Remove and reserve.

3. Sauté onion and garlic in oil in skillet 3 minutes. Add green pepper, tomatoes, currants, and thyme. Bring to a boil. Return chicken to skillet; reduce heat. Cover and simmer until chicken is tender, about 15 minutes, spooning juices over occasionally. Sprinkle with almonds, if desired.

Method-Microwave

1. Brush chicken with oil; sprinkle with curry powder, salt, if desired, and red pepper.
2. Place in 11-by-7-inch microwave-safe casserole dish with meaty portions toward outer edges of casserole. Cover with waxed paper. Cook on high power 8 minutes, turning chicken over after 4 minutes.
3. Remove chicken and reserve. Toss onion and garlic in drippings in casserole dish. Cover with waxed paper; cook on high power 3 minutes. Stir in green pepper, tomatoes, currants, and thyme. Cover with waxed paper; bring to a boil on high power, about 5 minutes. Return chicken to casserole, spooning juices over. Cover with waxed paper; cook on high power until chicken is tender, about 10–12 minutes, rotating dish once. Sprinkle with almonds, if desired.

Note: Legend has it that this recipe originated in Savannah, Georgia, from a sea captain selling spices.

Deep South Barbecued Chicken

		Nutrient Content per Serving		
Yield: 6 servings				
Serving Size: ⅙ recipe		CAL 181	Na	181 (mg)
Exchanges:		PRO 25 (gm)	K	324 (mg)
Meat, lean	3.0	Fat 6.4 (gm)	Fiber	0 (gm)
Vegetable	1.0	CHO 5 (gm)	Chol	75 (mg)

Ingredients

¼ CUP NO-SALT-ADDED TOMATO PASTE
1 TABLESPOON BROWN SUGAR
1 TABLESPOON REDUCED-SODIUM SOY SAUCE
1 TABLESPOON GRATED ONION
½ TEASPOON FRESHLY GROUND BLACK PEPPER
3 POUND BROILER-FRYER CHICKEN, CUT UP AND
SKINNED (2¾ POUNDS AFTER SKINNING)

Method

1. Combine tomato paste, sugar, soy sauce, onion, and pepper; mix well. (Mixture will be thick.)
2. Grill or broil chicken pieces 7–8 inches from heat source 15 minutes, turning once. Brush lightly with sauce; continue to cook 10–15 minutes or until chicken is tender, turning and brushing with sauce until sauce is used up.

Method-Microwave

1. Prepare sauce as directed in step 1 above.
2. Place chicken in 11-by-7-inch microwave-safe baking dish with meaty portions toward outer edges of dish. Cover with waxed paper; cook on high power 5 minutes. Turn chicken over; cover with waxed paper and continue to cook 5 minutes. Brush half of sauce over chicken. Cover with waxed paper; cook on high power 2–3 minutes. Turn chicken over; brush with remaining sauce. Cover with waxed paper and continue to cook on high power 2–3 minutes or until chicken is tender. Let stand 3 minutes.

Low-Fat Oven-Fried Chicken

Yield: 6 servings
Serving Size: ⅙ recipe
Exchanges:
Starch/Bread   0.5
Meat, lean   3.0

Nutrient Content per Serving

CAL	181	*Na	150 (mg)
PRO	25 (gm)	K	297 (mg)
Fat	5.3 (gm)	Fiber	0.5 (gm)
CHO	7 (gm)	Chol	62 (mg)

*Add 178 mg if optional salt is used.

Ingredients

    1 CUP PLAIN LOW-FAT YOGURT
    1 TEASPOON PAPRIKA
    1 TEASPOON THYME LEAVES
    ½ TEASPOON SALT (OPTIONAL)
    ¼ TEASPOON CAYENNE PEPPER
    ¼ TEASPOON GARLIC POWDER
    2 POUNDS CHICKEN THIGHS AND/OR BONELESS
       BREASTS, SKINNED
       NONSTICK VEGETABLE SPRAY
    1 CUP WHOLE WHEAT BREAD CRUMBS
    1 TABLESPOON MARGARINE, MELTED

Method

1. Heat oven to 400°F.
2. Combine yogurt, paprika, thyme, if desired, salt, pepper, and garlic powder; mix well. Coat chicken with mixture. Chicken may be covered and refrigerated overnight or until baking, or baked immediately.
3. Spray shallow roasting pan or jelly-roll pan with vegetable spray. Combine bread crumbs and margarine in shallow dish, mixing well. Coat chicken in crumbs; place in pan. Bake breasts 25 minutes, thighs 30–35 minutes or until chicken is tender and juices run clear.

Chicken in Saffron Cream Sauce

Yield: 6 servings

Serving Size: ⅙ recipe

Exchanges:

Meat, lean   3.0

Vegetable   1.0

Nutrient Content per Serving

CAL	171	*Na	73 (mg)
PRO	23 (gm)	K	212 (mg)
Fat	5.6 (gm)	Fiber	0.6 (gm)
CHO	5 (gm)	Chol	60 (mg)

*Add 178 mg if optional salt is used.

Ingredients

1 MEDIUM ONION, CHOPPED

2 CLOVES GARLIC, MINCED

1 TABLESPOON OLIVE OIL

2 TABLESPOONS ALL-PURPOSE FLOUR

½ CUP REDUCED-SODIUM CHICKEN BROTH OR HOMEMADE (PAGE 118)

¼ CUP DRY WHITE WINE OR VERMOUTH

1 TABLESPOON CHOPPED FRESH THYME OR 1 TEA-SPOON DRIED THYME

½ TEASPOON SALT (OPTIONAL)

¼ TEASPOON POWDERED SAFFRON

2 POUNDS CHICKEN THIGHS AND/OR SMALL BONE-LESS BREASTS, SKINNED

¼ CUP DAIRY SOUR HALF-AND-HALF (LITE SOUR CREAM)

2 TABLESPOONS CHOPPED FRESH PARSLEY OR CILANTRO

Method

1. Sauté onion and garlic in oil in 10-inch skillet until tender, about 4 minutes. Sprinkle with flour; cook and stir 1 minute. Add broth, wine, thyme, salt, if desired, and saffron; mix well. Add chicken, spooning sauce over. Cover and simmer

over low heat until chicken is tender, about 30 minutes, turning occasionally.
2. Remove chicken to serving platter. Remove skillet from heat; stir in sour cream until well blended. Pour over chicken; sprinkle with parsley.

Method-Microwave

1. Toss onion and garlic with oil in 11-by-7-inch microwave-safe baking dish. Cover and cook on high power 3 minutes. Stir in flour. Add broth, wine, thyme, salt, if desired, and saffron; mix well. Place chicken meaty side down in dish; spoon sauce over. Cover with vented plastic wrap and cook 12 minutes. Turn chicken over placing thicker portions toward outside of dish. Cover with vented plastic wrap and continue to cook on high power 8–10 minutes, or until chicken is tender.
2. Remove chicken to serving platter. Stir sour cream into sauce until well blended; pour over chicken. Sprinkle with parsley.

Note: Saffron is a very expensive spice, but just a little gives this dish a very lovely, heady flavor. If purchasing saffron threads (found in vials in specialty stores or large supermarkets), crush enough to equal ¼ teaspoon for this recipe. Serve with rice or pasta (not included in nutrient content) and spoon some of the sauce over.

Brunswick Stew

Yield: 6 servings
Serving Size: ⅙ recipe
Exchanges:

		Nutrient Content per Serving			
		CAL	272	Na	113 (mg)
		PRO	27 (gm)	K	714 (mg)
Starch/Bread	1.0	Fat	8.1 (gm)	Fiber	2.6 (gm)
Meat, lean	3.0	CHO	24 (gm)	Chol	67 (mg)
Vegetable	1.0				

Ingredients

3-POUND BROILER-FRYER CHICKEN, CUT UP AND
SKINNED
2 TABLESPOONS ALL-PURPOSE FLOUR
½ TEASPOON FRESHLY GROUND BLACK PEPPER
1 TABLESPOON OLIVE OIL
1 LARGE ONION, CHOPPED
1 28-OUNCE CAN NO-SALT-ADDED TOMATOES,
UNDRAINED AND COARSELY CHOPPED
1 CUP FROZEN WHOLE KERNEL CORN, THAWED
1 CUP FROZEN BABY LIMA BEANS, THAWED
1 SMALL JALAPEÑO PEPPER, SEEDED AND FINELY
CHOPPED (OPTIONAL)

Method

1. Dredge chicken pieces in flour combined with pepper. Brown in oil in large, deep skillet or Dutch oven.
2. Add onion, cook 1 minute. Stir in tomatoes; bring to a boil. Reduce heat; cover and simmer 20–30 minutes.
3. Stir in corn, lima beans, and jalapeño pepper, if desired. Cover and continue to simmer until vegetables are tender, about 15 minutes.

Method-Microwave

1. Place chicken and onion in 3-quart microwave-safe casserole dish. Sprinkle with flour and pepper; drizzle with oil. Cover with waxed paper; cook on high power 5 minutes.

2. Add tomatoes. Cover tightly and cook on high power 15–20 minutes or until chicken is tender, rotating dish and turning chicken over after 10 minutes.
3. Stir in corn and lima beans; continue to cook covered on high power 6–8 minutes or until vegetables are tender.

Herb and Garlic Grilled Chicken

Yield: 4 servings
Serving Size: ¼ recipe
Exchanges:
Meat, lean   3.0

Nutrient Content per Serving

CAL	164	Na	63 (mg)
PRO	26 (gm)	K	222 (mg)
Fat	5.5 (gm)	Fiber	0 (gm)
CHO	0 (gm)	Chol	72 (mg)

Ingredients

1 TABLESPOON OLIVE OIL
2 CLOVES GARLIC, MINCED
1 TABLESPOON EACH CHOPPED FRESH TARRAGON, ROSEMARY, THYME, OREGANO, AND MINT LEAVES (OR SUBSTITUTE 1 TEASPOON EACH DRIED)
½ TEASPOON FRESHLY GROUND BLACK PEPPER
2 WHOLE CHICKEN BREASTS, SPLIT, BONED, AND SKINNED (1 POUND)

Method

1. Combine oil, garlic, herbs, and pepper in shallow dish or plastic bag. Add chicken; turn to coat. Cover and refrigerate at least 6 hours or overnight.
2. Grill or broil chicken 6–8 inches from heat source 5–6 minutes per side or until chicken is tender, basting frequently with remaining herb mixture.

Chicken in Plum Tomatoes

Yield: 4 servings
Serving Size: ¼ recipe
Exchanges:

		Nutrient Content per Serving			
		CAL	211	*Na	189 (mg)
		PRO	28 (gm)	K	462 (mg)
Meat, lean	3.0	Fat	6.7 (gm)	Fiber	1.6 (gm)
Vegetable	2.0	CHO	9 (gm)	Chol	72 (mg)

*Add 133 mg if optional salt is used.

Ingredients

2 WHOLE CHICKEN BREASTS, SPLIT, BONED, AND SKINNED
1 TABLESPOON ALL-PURPOSE FLOUR
1 TEASPOON ROSEMARY, CRUSHED
¼ TEASPOON SALT (OPTIONAL)
¼ TEASPOON FRESHLY GROUND BLACK PEPPER
1 TABLESPOON OLIVE OIL
1 LARGE ONION, CUT INTO THIN WEDGES
1 CLOVE GARLIC, MINCED
1 TABLESPOON BALSAMIC OR RED WINE VINEGAR
1 16-OUNCE CAN ITALIAN PLUM TOMATOES, DRAINED AND HALVED
1 TEASPOON SUGAR

Method

1. Sprinkle chicken with flour, rosemary, salt, if desired, and pepper. Heat oil in large nonstick skillet over medium heat. Sauté onion and garlic until tender, about 4 minutes; push to edges of skillet. Add chicken; brown on both sides, about 6 minutes.
2. Deglaze pan with vinegar, then add tomatoes and sugar. Cover; cook 5 minutes or until chicken is tender.

Method-Microwave

1. Sprinkle chicken with rosemary, salt, if desired, and pepper.
   Toss oil, onion, and garlic in 1½-quart shallow microwave-
   safe casserole dish or 10-inch glass pie plate. Cover; cook on
   high power 4 minutes. Lay chicken over vegetables; cover
   and cook on high power 4 minutes.
2. Turn chicken over; add tomatoes, flour, vinegar, and sugar.
   Cover and cook on high power 6–8 minutes or until chicken is
   tender. Remove chicken to warm serving plate. Stir vegetables; cook uncovered on high power 3–4 minutes, until
   thickened.

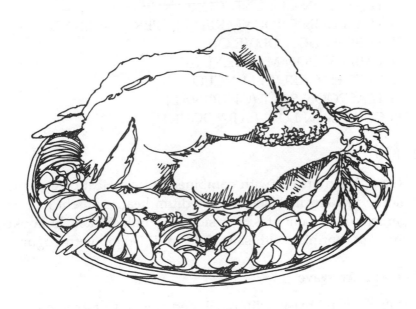

Indian Spiced Chicken Breasts

YIELD: 4 servings
Serving Size: ¼ recipe
Exchanges:
Meat, lean   3.5

Nutrient Content per Serving

CAL	208	*Na	107 (mg)
PRO	27 (gm)	K	262 (mg)
Fat	9.5 (gm)	Fiber	0 (gm)
CHO	2 (gm)	Chol	73 (mg)

*Add 133 mg if optional salt is used.

Ingredients

    2 WHOLE CHICKEN BREASTS, SPLIT, BONED, AND
    SKINNED
    1 TEASPOON GROUND CUMIN
    1 TEASPOON PAPRIKA
    ½ TEASPOON TURMERIC
    ½ TEASPOON GROUND CORIANDER
    ¼ TEASPOON GROUND RED PEPPER (CAYENNE)
    1 TABLESPOON OLIVE OIL
    1 TABLESPOON MARGARINE
    2 CLOVES GARLIC, MINCED
    ¼ TEASPOON SALT (OPTIONAL)
    ¼ CUP PLAIN LOW-FAT YOGURT

Method

1. Rub chicken breasts with combined spices. Heat oil and margarine in 10-inch skillet over medium heat. Add chicken and garlic; cook 5 minutes per side or until chicken is cooked through. Sprinkle with salt, if desired. Dollop with yogurt.

Method-Microwave

1. Rub chicken breasts with combined spices. Combine oil, margarine, and garlic in shallow microwave-safe casserole dish large enough to hold chicken in one layer. Cook on high until margarine is melted, about 40 seconds. Place chicken in dish; turn to coat. Cover with waxed paper and cook on high

power 3 minutes. Turn chicken over and continue to cook covered with waxed paper 3–5 minutes or until chicken is tender. Let stand covered 2 minutes. Sprinkle with salt, if desired. Dollop with yogurt.

Warm Sesame Chicken Salad

Yield: 4 servings
Serving Size: ¼ recipe
Exchanges:

Meat, lean	4.0
Vegetable	1.0
Fat	1.0

Nutrient Content per Serving

CAL	296	*Na	174 (mg)
PRO	30 (gm)	K	350 (mg)
Fat	15.5 (gm)	Fiber	1.2 (gm)
CHO	8 (gm)	Chol	72 (mg)

*Add 266 mg if optional salt is used.

Ingredients

    1 EGG WHITE
    1 TABLESPOON WATER
    ⅓ CUP DRY BREAD CRUMBS
    2 TABLESPOONS TOASTED SESAME SEEDS
    ½ TEASPOON PAPRIKA
    ½ TEASPOON SALT (OPTIONAL)
    2 WHOLE CHICKEN BREASTS, SPLIT, BONED, AND
        SKINNED (1 POUND)
    1 TABLESPOON MARGARINE
    2 CUPS ASSORTED TORN GREENS SUCH AS CHICORY,
        RED LEAF LETTUCE, OR ROMAINE
    2 TABLESPOONS PEANUT OR VEGETABLE OIL
    1 TABLESPOON FRESH LEMON JUICE
    1 TEASPOON ORIENTAL SESAME OIL (OPTIONAL)
        LEMON WEDGES

(continued on page 224)

Method

1. Beat egg white with water in shallow dish. Combine bread crumbs, sesame seeds, paprika, and salt in another shallow dish. Dip chicken in egg mixture; then in crumbs to coat, patting well.
2. Heat margarine in 10-inch nonstick skillet over medium-high heat. Sauté chicken in skillet until tender, about 5 minutes per side.
3. Combine peanut oil, lemon juice, and sesame oil, if desired. Toss with greens. Divide among 4 salad plates; top with chicken. Serve with lemon wedges.

Method-Microwave

1. Prepare chicken as in step 1 above.
2. Place in shallow 2-quart microwave-safe casserole dish. Melt margarine; drizzle over chicken. Cover with paper towel; cook on high power 6–8 minutes or until tender, turning chicken over after 4 minutes. Let stand covered 2 minutes.
3. Prepare and serve salad as in step 3 above.

Fish and Seafood

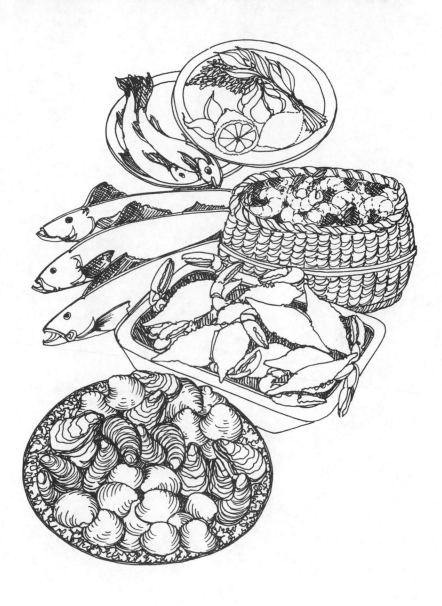

Cajun Grilled Red Snapper

Yield: 2 servings
Serving Size: ½ recipe
Exchanges:
Meat, lean   3.0

Nutrient Content per Serving

CAL	131	Na	316 (mg)
PRO	23 (gm)	K	462 (mg)
Fat	3.8 (gm)	Fiber	0 (gm)
CHO	0 (gm)	Chol	40 (mg)

Ingredients

    2 RED SNAPPER OR OTHER FIRM, WHITE FISH FILLETS,
        4 OUNCES EACH
    1 TEASPOON OLIVE OIL
    ¼ TEASPOON SALT
    1 GARLIC CLOVE
    ½ TEASPOON CRACKED BLACK PEPPER
    ½ TEASPOON THYME OR OREGANO, DRIED
    ¼ TEASPOON CAYENNE PEPPER
    ¼ TEASPOON GROUND WHITE PEPPER
        LEMON WEDGES

Method

1. Brush snapper evenly with oil. Sprinkle with combined seasonings.
2. Grill covered over medium coals or broil 6 inches from heat source 4–5 minutes per side or until fish is firm and opaque. Serve with lemon wedges.

Marinated Marlin

Yield: 4 servings
Serving Size: 4 ounces fish
Exchanges:
Meat, lean   3.0

Nutrient Content per Serving

CAL	169	*Na	103 (mg)
PRO	22 (gm)	K	345 (mg)
Fat	8 (gm)	Fiber	0 (gm)
CHO	1 (gm)	Chol	43 (mg)

*Add 133 mg if optional salt is used.

Ingredients

> 2 TABLESPOONS DRY VERMOUTH
> 1 TABLESPOON OLIVE OIL
> ¼ CUP CHOPPED GREEN ONIONS WITH TOPS
> 2 TABLESPOONS CHOPPED FRESH BASIL OR 2
>   TEASPOONS DRIED
> 1 CLOVE GARLIC, MINCED
> ½ TEASPOON DRIED MARJORAM
> ¼ TEASPOON RED PEPPER FLAKES
> ¼ TEASPOON SALT (OPTIONAL)
> 1 POUND MARLIN, SWORDFISH, TUNA, OR HALIBUT
>   STEAKS, CUT ¾ TO 1 INCH THICK
>   LEMON OR LIME WEDGES

Method

1. Combine vermouth, oil, green onions, basil, garlic, marjoram, pepper flakes, and salt. Pour over marlin.
2. Cover and refrigerate 1–2 hours.
3. Grill covered over medium coals or broil 6 inches from heat source 4–5 minutes per side or until fish is firm and opaque, basting with marinade. Do not overcook or fish will be tough and dry. Serve with lemon wedges.

Method-Microwave

1. Marinate marlin as directed above in shallow 2-quart microwave-safe dish.

2. Cover with vented plastic wrap. Cook on high power 2 minutes. Turn marlin over; cover and cook on high power 2–3 minutes or until fish is opaque.
3. Let stand covered 2 minutes. Serve with lemon wedges.

Note: Fish that are darker in color, such as tuna and marlin, are high in the fatty acid Omega 3. Take care not to overcook this type of fish or it will become very tough.

Spicy Fish Stew

Yield: 8 cups (8 servings)
Serving Size: 1 cup
Exchanges:
Meat, lean   1.0
Vegetable   3.0

Nutrient Content per Serving

CAL	133	Na	89 (mg)
PRO	17 (gm)	K	715 (mg)
Fat	2.2 (gm)	Fiber	2 (gm)
CHO	11 (gm)	Chol	37 (mg)

Ingredients

    8 OUNCES MUSHROOMS, SLICED
    1 CUP SLICED CELERY
    1 CUP CHOPPED ONION
    1 CLOVE GARLIC, MINCED
    2 TEASPOONS OLIVE OIL
    1 TEASPOON THYME
    1 TEASPOON SUGAR
    4 CUPS NO-SALT-ADDED TOMATO JUICE OR VEGETABLE JUICE COCKTAIL
    1 BAY LEAF
    ½ TEASPOON HOT PEPPER SAUCE
    ½ TEASPOON FRESHLY GROUND BLACK PEPPER
    1 POUND FIRM, WHITE FISH FILLETS SUCH AS SCROD, COD, OR PERCH, CUT INTO 1-INCH PIECES
    ¼ CUP CHOPPED PARSLEY

(continued on page 230)

Method

1. Sauté mushrooms, celery, onion, and garlic in oil in large saucepan over medium heat 3 minutes until tender.
2. Add thyme and sugar; sauté 1 minute. Add tomato juice, bay leaf, pepper sauce, and pepper; bring to a boil.
3. Reduce heat; add fish and simmer uncovered 10 minutes.
4. Discard bay leaf; stir in parsley. Ladle into soup bowls.

Method-Microwave

1. Toss mushrooms, celery, onion, and garlic with oil in 2½-quart round microwave-safe casserole. Cover and cook on high power 6 minutes, stirring once.
2. Stir in thyme, sugar, tomato juice, bay leaf, pepper sauce, and pepper. Cover and cook on high power until boiling, about 5–7 minutes.
3. Stir in fish; cover and cook on medium power 8–10 minutes, stirring once.
4. Discard bay leaf; stir in parsley. Ladle into soup bowls.

Fish and Vegetable Kabobs

Yield: 4 servings
Serving Size: ¼ recipe
Exchanges:
Meat, lean   3.0
Vegetable   1.0

Nutrient Content per Serving

CAL	178	Na	108 (mg)
PRO	23 (gm)	K	529 (mg)
Fat	7.1 (gm)	Fiber	2.6 (gm)
CHO	5 (gm)	Chol	44 (mg)

Ingredients

1 POUND MONKFISH OR SWORDFISH, CUT INTO 1–1½-INCH PIECES

1 SMALL JAPANESE EGGPLANT, CUT INTO ½-INCH SLICES (3–4 OUNCES)

1 MEDIUM ZUCCHINI OR YELLOW SQUASH, CUT INTO ½-INCH SLICES (4 OUNCES)

1 LARGE RED BELL PEPPER, CUT INTO 1-INCH PIECES
(6 OUNCES)
3 LARGE GREEN ONIONS WITH TOPS, CUT INTO
1½-INCH PIECES (2 OUNCES)
2 TABLESPOONS VERMOUTH OR DRY WHITE WINE
2 TABLESPOONS LEMON JUICE
2 TEASPOONS OLIVE OIL
2 TEASPOONS DILL OR TARRAGON
1 TEASPOON DRY MUSTARD
½ TEASPOON FRESHLY GROUND BLACK PEPPER

Method

1. Alternately thread fish, eggplant, squash, and bell pepper, with 1 piece of green onion between each, onto skewers. Place on shallow dish.
2. Combine vermouth, lemon juice, oil, dill, mustard, and pepper; mix well. Brush evenly over kabobs; let stand while heating coals or broiler.
3. Grill covered over medium coals or broil 6 inches from heat source 5 minutes per side or until fish is opaque and vegetables are crisp-tender, brushing with any marinade from dish.

Note: Japanese eggplant is available in Oriental markets and supermarkets with large produce departments. The shape is perfect for kabobs; however, regular eggplant may be substituted. Slice ½ inch thick, then cut into pieces to equal squash pieces.

Sashimi-Style Tuna Steaks

Yield: 2 servings
Serving Size: ½ recipe
Exchanges:
Meat, lean   3.0

Nutrient Content per Serving

CAL	168	Na	243 (mg)
PRO	26 (gm)	K	291 (mg)
Fat	6.2 (gm)	Fiber	0 (gm)
CHO	1 (gm)	Chol	42 (mg)

Ingredients

     1 8-OUNCE FRESH TUNA STEAK, CUT 1 INCH THICK
     1 TABLESPOON RICE WINE OR VERMOUTH
     2 TEASPOONS REDUCED-SODIUM SOY SAUCE
     1 TEASPOON ORIENTAL SESAME OIL
     1 SMALL CLOVE GARLIC, MINCED
     ¼ TEASPOON CRACKED SZECHUAN PEPPERCORNS OR
     RED PEPPER FLAKES

Method

1. Place tuna in shallow glass plate or dish.
2. Combine remaining ingredients; mix well.
3. Pour over tuna. Cover and refrigerate 1–2 hours.
4. Grill uncovered over hot coals or broil 5–6 inches from heat source 3 minutes per side or until tuna is firm but rare in center. Do not overcook.
5. Slice into thin strips; fan out on hot plates. Serve immediately.

Whitefish with Cilantro Pesto

Yield: 2 servings
Serving Size: 1 4-ounce fillet
Exchanges:
Meat, lean   3.0
Fat   0.5

Nutrient Content per Serving

CAL	197	Na	60 (mg)
PRO	22 (gm)	K	417 (mg)
Fat	11.3 (gm)	Fiber	0 (gm)
CHO	1 (gm)	Chol	68 (mg)

Ingredients

2 WHITEFISH, SCROD, SOLE, OR FLOUNDER FILLETS,
ABOUT 4 OUNCES EACH
1 TABLESPOON LEMON OR LIME JUICE
1 CLOVE GARLIC
1 CUP CILANTRO LEAVES, STEMS REMOVED
2 TEASPOONS OLIVE OIL
¼ TEASPOON SALT
¼ TEASPOON RED PEPPER FLAKES OR ⅛ TEASPOON
CAYENNE PEPPER
LEMON OR LIME WEDGES

Method

1. Heat oven to 400°F. Place fish in shallow baking dish; sprinkle with lemon juice.
2. Mince garlic in food processor fitted with steel blade. Add cilantro; process until minced. Add oil, salt, and pepper flakes; process until well mixed. (Or mince garlic and cilantro by hand; stir in oil, salt, and pepper until well blended.)
3. Spread evenly over fish. Bake 10 minutes or until fish is opaque and firm. Serve with lemon wedges.

Method-Microwave

1. Place fish in shallow microwave-safe dish; sprinkle with lemon juice.
2. Prepare cilantro pesto as directed in step 2 above.
3. Spread evenly over fish. Cover with vented plastic wrap. Cook on high power 3–4 minutes, rotating dish once. Let stand covered 3 minutes. Serve with lemon wedges.

Halibut with Mustard Seeds

Yield: 2 servings
Serving Size: ½ recipe
Exchanges:
Meat, lean   3.0

Nutrient Content per Serving

CAL	159	Na	107 (mg)
PRO	24 (gm)	K	514 (mg)
Fat	6.3 (gm)	Fiber	0 (gm)
CHO	0 (gm)	Chol	37 (mg)

Ingredients

8 OUNCES HALIBUT, SCROD, OR GROUPER FILLETS
2 TEASPOONS CRUSHED MUSTARD SEEDS
HUNGARIAN PAPRIKA, PREFERABLY HOT
(OPTIONAL)
2 TEASPOONS MARGARINE
1½ TABLESPOONS LEMON JUICE

Method

1. Sprinkle halibut evenly with mustard seeds; press in. If desired, sprinkle lightly with hot paprika.
2. Melt margarine in large nonstick skillet over medium heat. Add halibut; sauté until opaque and firm, about 3–4 minutes per side depending on thickness of fillet.
3. Remove halibut to warm serving platter. Add lemon juice to skillet; stir well and pour juices over halibut.

Method-Microwave

1. Prepare halibut as in step 1 above.
2. Place margarine in shallow microwave-safe dish. Cook on high power until melted, about 45 seconds.
3. Stir in lemon juice. Add halibut, turn to coat. Cover with vented plastic wrap. Cook on high power 4–5 minutes or until fish is opaque and firm, rotating dish once.

Wisconsin-Style Fish Boil

Yield: 4 servings
Serving Size: ¼ recipe
Exchanges:
Starch/Bread 1.0
Meat, lean 4.0
Vegetable 1.0

Nutrient Content per Serving
CAL 331 Na 222 (mg)
PRO 36 (gm) K 1201 (mg)
Fat 10.5 (gm) Fiber 4.4 (gm)
CHO 23 (gm) Chol 102 (mg)

Ingredients

    2 CUPS WATER
    1 CUP CLAM JUICE
    1 MEDIUM CARROT, CHOPPED
    1 MEDIUM ONION, CHOPPED
    2 STALKS CELERY, CHOPPED
    3 PARSLEY SPRIGS OR CELERY TOPS
    2 TEASPOONS WHOLE PEPPERCORNS
    1 POUND RED POTATOES, UNPEELED AND HALVED
      IF SMALL, QUARTERED IF LARGE
    4 SMALL YELLOW ONIONS, PEELED AND QUARTERED
      (8 OUNCES)
    4 LAKE TROUT, WHITEFISH, OR COHO SALMON
      STEAKS (1½ POUNDS)
      MINCED PARSLEY
      LEMON WEDGES

Method

1. Combine water, clam juice, carrot, onion, celery, parsley sprigs, and peppercorns in large saucepan or Dutch oven. Bring to a boil; reduce heat. Cover and simmer 20 minutes. Strain and discard vegetables.
2. Return broth to pan. Add potatoes and onions; bring to a boil. Cover and simmer 17–20 minutes or until potatoes are tender.

(continued on page 236)

3. Add fish; simmer until fish is opaque, about 6–7 minutes. With slotted spoon, divide fish, potatoes, and onions into 4 bowls. Ladle ⅓ cup broth into each bowl. Sprinkle with parsley; serve with lemon.

Method-Microwave

1. Combine water, clam juice, carrot, onion, celery, parsley sprigs, and peppercorns in 3-quart microwave-safe casserole dish. Cover and cook on high power until boiling, about 8 minutes. Reduce power to medium and continue cooking 15 minutes. Strain and discard vegetables.
2. Return broth to dish. Add potatoes and onions; cook on high power until boiling, about 4 minutes. Reduce power to medium and continue to cook 15–20 minutes or until potatoes are tender.
3. Add fish; cover and cook at high power 1 minute. Reduce power to medium and continue to cook until fish is opaque, about 7–9 minutes. With slotted spoon, divide fish, potatoes, and onions among 4 bowls. Ladle ⅓ cup broth into each bowl. Sprinkle with parsley; serve with lemon.

Note: This dish is typically served in Door County, Wisconsin. A huge cauldron is set over an open flame outdoors and guests watch as the huge quantities of ingredients are lowered into the boiling seasoned water in strainers. This broth is so flavorful that you won't miss the generous ladle of butter traditionally poured on at the end.

Baked Salmon with Horseradish Mayonnaise

Yield: 4 servings	Nutrient Content per Serving			
Serving Size: ¼ recipe	CAL	229	Na	124 (mg)
Exchanges:	PRO	25 (gm)	K	378 (mg)
Meat, lean 4.0	Fat	12.5 (gm)	Fiber	1 (gm)
	CHO	3 (gm)	Chol	81 (mg)

Ingredients

    NONSTICK VEGETABLE SPRAY
    1 POUND SALMON FILLETS IN 4 SERVING PIECES
    2 TABLESPOONS FINELY CHOPPED SHALLOTS
    ¼ CUP DRY WHITE WINE OR VERMOUTH
    2 TABLESPOONS REDUCED-CALORIE MAYONNAISE
    2 TABLESPOONS REDUCED-CALORIE SOUR CREAM
    2 TEASPOONS LEMON JUICE
  2–3 TEASPOONS FRESHLY GRATED HORSERADISH OR
    DRAINED, PREPARED HORSERADISH
    2 TEASPOONS RINSED AND DRAINED CAPERS
    (OPTIONAL)

Method

1. Preheat oven to 450°F.
2. Spray shallow roasting pan or baking dish with vegetable spray. Place fillets, skin side down, into pan.
3. Sprinkle shallots over fillets; pour wine evenly over all. Bake 6–8 minutes or just until fish is opaque.
4. Combine mayonnaise, sour cream, lemon juice, and horseradish; mix well.
5. Transfer salmon to warm serving plates with slotted spatula, discarding shallots; dollop with mayonnaise. Garnish with capers, if desired.

Method-Microwave

1. Spray shallow microwave-safe baking dish with vegetable cooking spray. Place fillets, skin side down, into dish.
2. Sprinkle shallots over fillets; pour wine evenly over all. Cover with vented plastic wrap. Cook on high power 4–5 minutes or just until fish is opaque, rotating dish once. Let stand covered 2 minutes.
3. Prepare mayonnaise and serve fish as directed in steps 4 and 5 above.

Note: The salmon may also be served at room temperature, which makes for good picnic fare. Be sure to keep the horseradish mayonnaise chilled.

Salmon with Grapefruit

Yield: 2 servings	Nutrient Content per Serving			
Serving Size: ½ recipe	CAL	256	Na	68 (mg)
Exchanges:	PRO	28 (gm)	K	452 (mg)
Meat, lean 4.0	Fat	13.6 (gm)	Fiber	0.5 (gm)
Fat 0.5	CHO	4 (gm)	Chol	89 (mg)

Ingredients

¼ CUP MINCED SHALLOTS OR SWEET ONION
1 TEASPOON SAFFLOWER OIL
1 LARGE SALMON FILLET (8 OUNCES)
¼ CUP FRESH GRAPEFRUIT JUICE, PREFERABLY PINK

Method

1. Sauté shallots in oil in small nonstick skillet until tender, about 4 minutes. Add salmon; pour grapefruit juice over. Cover and simmer over low heat until salmon is opaque, about 6–8 minutes.
2. Cut salmon into 2 serving-size portions; place on warmed plates. Increase heat under skillet and cook juices until bubbly; pour over salmon.

Shrimp Vera Cruz

Yield: 4 servings	Nutrient Content per Serving			
Serving Size: ¼ recipe	CAL	249	Na	240 (mg)
Exchanges:	PRO	19 (gm)	K	542 (mg)
Starch/Bread 2.0	Fat	2.7 (gm)	Fiber	2.8 (gm)
Meat, lean 1.0	CHO	37 (gm)	Chol	143 (mg)
Vegetable 2.0				

Ingredients

1 TEASPOON OLIVE OIl
1 MEDIUM ONION, CHOPPED (1 CUP)

2 GARLIC CLOVES, MINCED
1 14½-OUNCE CAN NO-SALT-ADDED STEWED
  TOMATOES
2 TEASPOONS CHOPPED FRESH JALAPEÑO PEPPER
  OR 1 TABLESPOON CHOPPED, PICKLED JALAPEÑO
  PEPPERS
1 SMALL GREEN OR RED BELL PEPPER, CUT INTO
  SHORT, THIN STRIPS (1 CUP)
1 POUND MEDIUM SHRIMP IN SHELL, PEELED AND
  DEVEINED (OR 12 OUNCES RAW SHRIMP, PEELED)
1 TABLESPOON CORNSTARCH MIXED WITH 1 TABLE-
  SPOON WATER
¼ CUP COARSELY CHOPPED CILANTRO
2 CUPS HOT COOKED BROWN RICE
  LIME WEDGES

Method

1. Heat oil in large nonstick skillet over medium heat. Sauté
   onion and garlic until tender, about 4 minutes. Add tomatoes
   and jalapeño pepper; simmer 10 minutes.
2. Add pepper strips and shrimp; cook until shrimp are opaque,
   about 5 minutes. Stir in cornstarch mixture; cook and stir
   until thickened, about 1 minute.
3. Stir in cilantro; serve over rice with lime wedges.

Method-Microwave

1. Combine oil, onion, and garlic in shallow 2-quart microwave-
   safe baking dish. Cover with vented plastic wrap; cook on
   high power 3 minutes. Add tomatoes and jalapeño pepper;
   cover and cook 6–7 minutes, rotating dish once.
2. Stir in pepper strips, shrimp, and cornstarch mixture; cover
   and cook 3–4 minutes, stirring once.
3. Serve as in step 3 above.

Gingered Sesame Scallops

Yield: 4 Servings	Nutrient Content per Serving		
Serving Size: ¼ recipe	CAL 107	Na	348 (mg)
Exchanges:	PRO 17 (gm)	K	366 (mg)
Meat, lean 2.0	Fat 3.3 (gm)	Fiber	0 (gm)
	CHO 1 (gm)	Chol	39 (mg)

Ingredients

        2 TEASPOONS ORIENTAL SESAME OIL
        1 POUND SEA OR BAY SCALLOPS, PATTED DRY
        2 CLOVES GARLIC, MINCED
¼–½ TEASPOON RED PEPPER FLAKES
        1 TABLESPOON REDUCED-SODIUM SOY SAUCE
        1 TABLESPOON SHREDDED FRESH GINGERROOT
        2 TABLESPOONS CHOPPED CILANTRO (OPTIONAL)

Method

1. Heat oil in nonstick skillet over medium-high heat.
2. Add scallops, garlic, and pepper flakes. Sauté until scallops are opaque and just cooked through, about 5 minutes for sea and 4 minutes for bay scallops.
3. Add soy sauce and ginger; cook and stir 1 minute or until liquid is absorbed. Sprinkle with cilantro.

Note: Fresh ginger keeps indefinitely in the freezer. It may be shredded in the frozen state without peeling, then returned to the freezer.

Fish Steaks Papillote

Yield: 2 servings
Serving Size: ½ recipe
Exchanges:
Meat, lean   4.0
Vegetable   1.0

Nutrient Content per Serving

CAL	246	*Na	201 (mg)
PRO	34 (gm)	K	532 (mg)
Fat	10.9 (gm)	Fiber	1 (gm)
CHO	1 (gm)	Chol	66 (mg)

*Add 267 mg if optional salt is used.

Ingredients

2 SWORDFISH, SALMON, TUNA, OR HALIBUT STEAKS
CUT ¾ INCH THICK (ABOUT ¾ POUND TOTAL)
2 TEASPOONS SUNFLOWER MARGARINE, MELTED
2 TEASPOONS LEMON OR LIME JUICE
2 TEASPOONS DRY WHITE WINE OR VERMOUTH
2 TEASPOONS CHOPPED FRESH TARRAGON OR DILL
OR ¾ TEASPOON DRIED TARRAGON OR DILL
¼ TEASPOON SALT (OPTIONAL)
¼ CUP RED BELL PEPPER STRIPS (1 OUNCE)
¼ CUP YELLOW BELL PEPPER STRIPS (1 OUNCE)
LEMON OR LIME WEDGES

Method

1. Cut 2 pieces heavy-duty or double-thickness aluminum foil into 12-inch squares. Place fish steaks on foil.
2. Combine margarine, lemon juice, wine, tarragon, salt, if desired, and pepper. Brush evenly over fish steaks; sprinkle with red and yellow pepper. Bring edges of foil together; seal tightly.
3. Place over medium coals or in preheated 400°F oven 5 minutes. Open foil; continue cooking 5–8 minutes or until fish is opaque. Serve with lemon wedges.

Barbecued Shrimp Kabobs

Yield: 4 servings	Nutrient Content per Serving			
Serving Size: ¼ recipe	CAL	137	*Na	204 (mg)
Exchanges:	PRO	18 (gm)	K	279 (mg)
Meat, lean 2.0	Fat	4.4 (gm)	Fiber	1 (gm)
Vegetable 1.0	CHO	5 (gm)	Chol	166 (mg)

*Add 133 mg if optional salt is used.

Ingredients

1 POUND LARGE SHRIMP, PEELED (WITH TAILS LEFT INTACT, IF DESIRED) AND DEVEINED
1 MEDIUM ONION, CUT INTO THIN WEDGES (6 OUNCES)
¼ CUP NO-SALT-ADDED CHILI SAUCE
1 TABLESPOON LEMON JUICE
1 TABLESPOON OLIVE OIL
1 CLOVE GARLIC, MINCED
½ TEASPOON ROSEMARY, CRUSHED
¼ TEASPOON HOT PEPPER SAUCE
¼ TEASPOON SALT (OPTIONAL)

Method

1. Place shrimp and onion wedges in shallow glass dish or plastic bag.
2. Combine remaining ingredients; pour over shrimp. Cover dish or tie bag securely and refrigerate at least 1 hour, turning once.
3. Drain shrimp and onions, reserving marinade. Alternately thread onto skewers.
4. Grill or broil 4–5 inches from heat source, turning and basting occasionally with marinade, until shrimp is opaque, about 6–8 minutes.

Lime-Grilled Fish with Fresh Salsa

Yield: 4 servings
Serving Size: ¼ recipe
Exchanges:
Meat, lean   3.0
Vegetable   1.0

Nutrient Content per Serving

CAL	161	*Na	57 (mg)
PRO	24 (gm)	K	646 (mg)
Fat	5.1 (gm)	Fiber	0.7 (gm)
CHO	4 (gm)	Chol	47 (mg)

*Add 133 mg if optional salt is used.

Ingredients

    1 LARGE TOMATO, SEEDED AND CHOPPED (8 OUNCES)
    ¼ CUP SLICED GREEN ONIONS
    ¼ CUP CHOPPED CILANTRO
    2 TABLESPOONS FRESH LIME JUICE, DIVIDED
    1 TABLESPOON CHOPPED JALAPEÑO PEPPER
    1 CLOVE GARLIC, MINCED
    ¼ TEASPOON SALT (OPTIONAL)
    1 TABLESPOON OLIVE OIL
    1 POUND FIRM FISH FILLETS SUCH AS ORANGE
    ROUGHY OR RED SNAPPER

Method

1. To make salsa, combine tomato, green onions, cilantro, 1 tablespoon of the lime juice, jalapeño pepper, garlic and salt, if desired. Cover and refrigerate until serving.
2. Combine oil and remaining lime juice; brush over fish. Grill or broil 4–5 inches from heat source until opaque, about 6 minutes, depending on thickness of fish. Serve immediately with salsa.

Method-Microwave

1. Prepare salsa as in step 1 above.
2. Combine oil and remaining lime juice; brush over fish. Place in shallow microwave-safe casserole dish. Cover with vented plastic wrap. Cook on high power 5–7 minutes or until fish is opaque, rotating dish once. Drain fish and serve immediately with salsa.

Stuffed Sole Fillets

Yield: 4 servings
Serving Size: 1 stuffed sole fillet
Exchanges:
Starch/Bread 0.5
Meat, lean 4.0

Nutrient Content per Serving

CAL	231	Na	165 (mg)
PRO	33 (gm)	K	546 (mg)
Fat	6.2 (gm)	Fiber	1.5 (gm)
CHO	9 (gm)	Chol	89 (mg)

Ingredients

1 SMALL ONION, FINELY CHOPPED (2 OUNCES)
1 CLOVE GARLIC, MINCED
2 TEASPOONS OLIVE OIL
⅓ CUP SHREDDED CARROT (1½ OUNCES, SMALL)
⅓ CUP SHREDDED ZUCCHINI OR YELLOW SQUASH (1½ OUNCES)
½ CUP COOKED WILD OR BROWN RICE (2 OUNCES)
2 TABLESPOONS CHOPPED ITALIAN OR REGULAR PARSLEY
⅛ TEASPOON FRESHLY GROUND BLACK PEPPER
4 SOLE FILLETS, 6 OUNCES EACH
2 TABLESPOONS DRY WHITE WINE
2 TEASPOONS MARGARINE, MELTED
1 TEASPOON SWEET HUNGARIAN PAPRIKA
LEMON WEDGES

Method

1. Preheat oven to 400°F.
2. Saute onion and garlic in oil until tender, about 4 minutes. Add carrot and zucchini; sauté 2 minutes. Add rice; sauté 1 minute. Remove from heat; stir in parsley and pepper.
3. Sprinkle sole with wine. Spoon rice mixture evenly down center of each fillet; roll up from short side. Place seam side down in shallow baking dish.
4. Brush with margarine; sprinkle with paprika. Bake 15–17 minutes or until fish is opaque and stuffing is hot. Serve with lemon wedges.

Method-Microwave

1. Toss onion and garlic with oil in shallow 2-quart microwave-safe casserole or 10-inch pie plate. Cover with waxed paper and cook on high power 2 minutes. Stir in carrot, zucchini, and rice; cover and cook 2 minutes. Stir in parsley and pepper.
2. Stuff fish as directed above in step 3. Place stuffed fish in same dish; cover with waxed paper. Cook on high power 6–8 minutes or until fish is opaque and stuffing is hot, rotating dish once during cooking. Serve with lemon wedges.

Fish Fillets in Red Pepper Purée

Yield: 4 servings
Serving Size: ¼ recipe

Exchanges:

| Meat, lean | 3.0 |
| Vegetable | 1.0 |

Nutrient Content per Serving

CAL	161	*Na	85 (mg)
PRO	24 (gm)	K	462 (mg)
Fat	3.3 (gm)	Fiber	3.8 (gm)
CHO	8 (gm)	Chol	56 (mg)

*Add 267 mg if optional salt is used.

Ingredients

    1 LARGE ONION, COARSELY CHOPPED (8 OUNCES)
    1 CLOVE GARLIC, MINCED
    2 TEASPOONS OLIVE OIL
    2 LARGE RED BELL PEPPERS, COARSELY CHOPPED (12 OUNCES)
    1 TEASPOON GROUND CORIANDER
⅛–¼ TEASPOON RED PEPPER FLAKES, AS DESIRED
    1 POUND FISH FILLETS SUCH AS SCROD, COD, HADDOCK, OR ORANGE ROUGHY
    ½ TEASPOON SALT (OPTIONAL)
    LIME WEDGES

(continued on page 246)

Method

1. Sauté onion and garlic in oil in 10-inch skillet until tender, about 5 minutes. Add red peppers, coriander, and pepper flakes; continue to sauté 1 minute. Cover and steam over low heat until peppers are very tender, 6–8 minutes.
2. Transfer to food processor fitted with steel blade; blend until smooth, scraping down sides twice. Stir in ¼ teaspoon salt, if desired.
3. Sprinkle fish with remaining salt, if desired. Place in same skillet. Spoon sauce on top of fish; cover and simmer until fish is opaque, about 8 minutes depending on thickness of fish. Remove with slotted spatula. Serve with lime wedges.

Method-Microwave

1. Combine onion, garlic, and oil in 2-quart microwave-safe baking dish. Cover and cook on high power 2 minutes. Add red peppers, coriander, and pepper flakes. Cover and cook until peppers are very tender, about 6 minutes, stirring once.
2. Transfer to food processor fitted with steel blade; process until smooth, scraping down sides twice. Stir in ¼ teaspoon salt, if desired.
3. Sprinkle fish with remaining salt, if desired. Place in same baking dish. Spoon sauce on top of fish; cover and cook on high power 5–7 minutes or until fish is opaque. Remove with slotted spatula. Serve with lime wedges.

Boston Scrod Dijon

Yield: 4 servings
Serving Size: ¼ recipe
Exchanges:
Meat, lean   2.0

Nutrient Content per Serving

CAL	115	Na	127 (mg)
PRO	20 (gm)	K	220 (mg)
Fat	1.9 (gm)	Fiber	0.1 (gm)
CHO	3 (gm)	Chol	49 (mg)

Ingredients

    1 POUND FRESH SCROD FILLETS, IN 4 SERVING-SIZE
      PIECES
    1 TABLESPOON REDUCED-CALORIE MAYONNAISE
    1 TEASPOON DIJON-SYTLE MUSTARD
    1 CLOVE GARLIC, MINCED
    2 TABLESPOONS DRY BREAD CRUMBS
      LEMON WEDGES

Method

1. Heat oven to 425°F.
2. Place fish in shallow ovenproof casserole dish in one layer.
   Combine mayonnaise, mustard, and garlic; spread over fish.
   Sprinkle with bread crumbs.
3. Bake fish 10–12 minutes or until opaque; serve with lemon
   wedges.

Method-Microwave

1. Place fish in microwave-safe casserole dish in one layer. Combine mayonnaise, mustard, and garlic; spread over fish. Sprinkle with bread crumbs.
2. Cook uncovered on high power 5–7 minutes or until fish is
   opaque, rotating dish once. Serve with lemon wedges.

New Hampshire Mussels in Broth

Yield: 4 servings	Nutrient Content per Serving		
Serving Size: ¼ recipe	CAL 117	Na	264 (mg)
Exchanges:	PRO 8 (gm)	K	215 (mg)
Meat, lean 1.0	Fat 7.3 (gm)	Fiber	0.2 (gm)
Vegetable 1.0	CHO 3 (gm)	Chol	18 (mg)
Fat 1.0			

Exchanges (rolls):	Nutrient Content per Serving		
Starch/Bread 1.5	CAL 114	Na	213 (mg)
	PRO 4 (gm)	K	43 (mg)
	Fat 1.3 (gm)	Fiber	0.8 (gm)
	CHO 21 (gm)	Chol	0 (mg)

Ingredients

- 2 POUNDS MUSSELS
- 2 TABLESPOONS MARGARINE
- ¼ CUP CHOPPED SHALLOT OR ONION
- 2 CLOVES GARLIC, MINCED
- ½ CUP DRY WHITE WINE
- ½ CUP REDUCED-SODIUM CHICKEN BROTH OR HOMEMADE (PAGE 118)
- ½ TEASPOON FRESHLY GROUND BLACK PEPPER
- 2 TABLESPOONS CHOPPED PARSLEY, PREFERABLY FLAT LEAF
- 4 SMALL HARD FRENCH ROLLS, HEATED (TOTAL OF 6 OUNCES)

Method

1. Soak mussels in cold water; rinse and scrape off beards.
2. In large deep skillet or sauté pan, melt margarine. Sauté shallot and garlic until tender, about 4 minutes.
3. Add wine, broth, and pepper; bring to a boil. Simmer uncovered 5 minutes. Add drained mussels; cover and cook until mussels are fully open, 8–10 minutes, shaking the pan frequently. Discard any mussels that do not open.

4. Ladle mussels and broth into soup bowls; sprinkle with parsley. Serve with rolls for dipping into broth, if desired.

Method-Microwave

1. Soak mussels in cold water; rinse and scrape off beards.
2. Place margarine in shallow microwave-safe casserole or baking dish that will hold mussels in one layer. Cook on high power until melted, about 45 seconds.
3. Toss shallot and garlic with margarine. Cover and cook on high power until tender, about 3 minutes. Stir in wine, broth, and pepper. Cook uncovered on high power 5 minutes. Add mussels; cover tightly and cook on high power until mussels are fully open, 7–9 minutes, rotating dish once. Discard any mussels that do not open.
4. Ladle mussels and broth into soup bowls; sprinkle with parsley. Serve with rolls for dipping into broth, if desired.

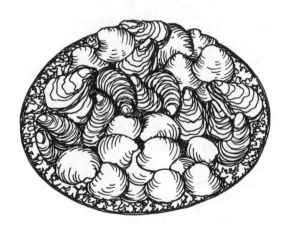

Gulf Coast Shrimp and Vegetables

Yield: 4 servings

Serving Size: ¼ recipe

Exchanges:

Meat, lean   2.0

Vegetable   1.0

Nutrient Content per Serving

CAL	133	*Na	192 (mg)
PRO	18 (gm)	K	306 (mg)
Fat	4.4 (gm)	Fiber	2.2 (gm)
CHO	5 (gm)	Chol	162 (mg)

*Add 133 mg if optional salt is used.

Ingredients

- 1 TABLESPOON OLIVE OIL
- 1 LARGE ONION, CUT INTO THIN WEDGES
- 1 SMALL RED BELL PEPPER, CUT INTO THIN STRIPS
- 2 CLOVES GARLIC, MINCED
- ¼ TEASPOON SALT (OPTIONAL)
- 1 POUND MEDIUM OR LARGE SHRIMP IN THE SHELL, PEELED AND DEVEINED (¾ POUND AFTER PEELING)
- 1 MEDIUM ZUCCHINI SQUASH, CUT INTO SHORT, THIN STRIPS
- 1 TABLESPOON CHOPPED FRESH THYME LEAVES OR 1 TEASPOON DRIED THYME
- ¼ TEASPOON RED PEPPER FLAKES

Method

1. Heat oil in large skillet over medium-high heat. Add onion, red pepper, and garlic. Sauté until limp, about 3 minutes. Sprinkle with salt, if desired.
2. Push onion mixture to edges of skillet. Add shrimp and zucchini; sprinkle with thyme and red pepper. Sauté until shrimp are opaque, 4–5 minutes.

Method-Microwave

1. Toss onion, red pepper, and garlic with oil in 11-by-7-inch microwave-safe baking dish. Cover and cook on high power 3 minutes. Sprinkle with salt, if desired.

2. Add shrimp and zucchini; sprinkle with thyme and red pepper. Cover and cook on high power 3–4 minutes, or until shrimp are opaque, stirring once.

Louisiana-Style Shrimp

		Nutrient Content per Serving		
Yield: 4 servings				
Serving Size: ¼ recipe		CAL 114	Na	188 (mg)
Exchanges:		PRO 18 (gm)	K	157 (mg)
Meat, lean	2.0	Fat 4.3 (gm)	Fiber	0 (gm)
		CHO 1 (gm)	Chol	162 (mg)

Ingredients

> 1 POUND MEDIUM OR LARGE SHRIMP, PEELED AND
> DEVEINED (¾ POUND AFTER PEELING)
> 1 TABLESPOON OLIVE OIL
> 2 CLOVES GARLIC, MINCED
> 1 TEASPOON CRUSHED DRIED ROSEMARY LEAVES
> 1 TEASPOON PAPRIKA
> ¼ TEASPOON GROUND RED PEPPER

Method

1. Heat oil in 10-inch nonstick skillet over medium heat. Add shrimp and garlic; sprinkle with remaining ingredients. Sauté until shrimp are opaque, 5–7 minutes depending on size. Serve immediately.

Method-Microwave

1. Toss shrimp and garlic with oil in 9- or 10-inch glass pie plate; sprinkle with remaining ingredients. Cover with waxed paper; cook on high power 3 minutes or until shrimp are opaque, stirring after each minute. Let stand, covered, 1 minute before serving.

Note: In Louisiana this dish is referred to as "barbecued shrimp," even though it is not grilled.

Chesapeake Oyster and Vegetable Stew

Yield: 6 servings

Serving Size: ⅙ recipe

Exchanges:

Starch/Bread	1.0
Meat, lean	1.0
Vegetable	1.0

Nutrient Content per Serving

CAL	151	*Na	153 (mg)
PRO	8 (gm)	K	598 (mg)
Fat	4.4 (gm)	Fiber	1.6 (gm)
CHO	21 (gm)	Chol	44 (mg)

*Add 178 mg if optional salt is used.

Ingredients

1 LARGE ONION, COARSELY CHOPPED
2 CLOVES GARLIC, MINCED
1 TABLESPOON OLIVE OIL
1 15½-OUNCE CAN NO-SALT-ADDED TOMATOES
2 CUPS DICED, PEELED POTATOES (½-INCH PIECES)
½ CUP DRY WHITE WINE
½ TEASPOON SALT (OPTIONAL)
½ TEASPOON FRESHLY GROUND BLACK PEPPER
½ TEASPOON DRIED THYME LEAVES
½ TEASPOON DRIED BASIL LEAVES
1 SMALL GREEN BELL PEPPER, DICED
1 SMALL RED BELL PEPPER, DICED
1 PINT SHUCKED OYSTERS, JUICES RESERVED
¼ CUP CHOPPED PARSLEY

Method

1. Sauté onion and garlic in oil in large saucepan until tender, about 4 minutes. Add tomatoes with liquid, potatoes, wine, salt (if desired), pepper, thyme, and basil. Cover and simmer until potatoes are tender, 20–24 minutes, stirring occasionally.
2. Add peppers and oysters with liquid; simmer uncovered until edges of oysters curl, 3–4 minutes. Ladle into shallow bowls; sprinkle with parsley.

Method-Microwave

1. Toss onion and garlic with oil in 3-quart microwave-safe casserole dish. Cover and cook on high power 4 minutes. Stir in tomatoes with liquid, potatoes, wine, salt (if desired), pepper, thyme, and basil. Cover and cook on high power 15–20 minutes or until potatoes are tender, stirring once.
2. Stir in peppers and oysters with liquid; cover and cook on high power 5–7 minutes or until edges of oysters curl. Ladle into shallow bowls; sprinkle with parsley.

Meatless
Main Dishes

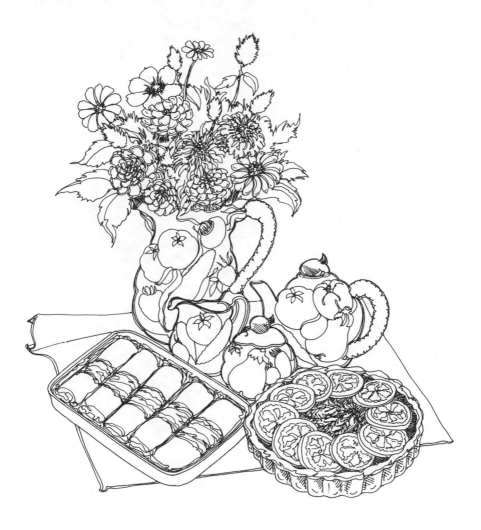

Florida Coast Rice with Beans

Yield: 4 main-dish servings
Serving Size: 1¼ cups
Exchanges:
Starch/Bread   4.0

Nutrient Content per Serving

CAL	312	Na	187 (mg)
PRO	11 (gm)	K	351 (mg)
Fat	3.3 (gm)	Fiber	6 (gm)
CHO	59 (gm)	Chol	0 (mg)

Ingredients

   1 CUP CHOPPED ONION
   1 CLOVE GARLIC, MINCED
   2 TEASPOONS OLIVE OIL
   1 CUP UNCOOKED RICE (PREFERABLY CONVERTED)
   1 CUP REDUCED-SODIUM CHICKEN BROTH
   1 CUP WATER
   ¼ CUP DRY WHITE WINE OR VERMOUTH
   1–2 TABLESPOONS CHOPPED JALAPEÑO PEPPERS,
      FRESH OR CANNED, DRAINED
   ⅛ TEASPOON GROUND CLOVES
   1 16-OUNCE CAN BLACK BEANS, RINSED AND DRAINED
   ⅓ CUP COARSELY CHOPPED CILANTRO
      LIME WEDGES

Method

1. Sauté onion and garlic in oil in large saucepan 2 minutes. Add rice; stir to coat.
2. Add broth, water, wine, peppers, and cloves. Bring to a boil. Reduce heat; cover and simmer until liquid is absorbed, about 20 minutes.
3. Stir in beans; heat through. Stir in cilantro. Serve with lime wedges.

Method-Microwave

1. Toss onion and garlic with oil in 2½-quart deep, microwave-safe casserole dish. Cover and cook on high power 2–3 minutes. Add rice; stir to coat.

(continued on page 258)

2. Reduce water to ¾ cup. Add broth, water, wine, peppers, and cloves. Cover and cook on high power until boiling, about 5–6 minutes. Reduce power to medium and continue to cook 17–18 minutes or until liquid is absorbed.
3. Stir in beans; cover and cook on high power 1 minute. Stir in cilantro. Serve with lime wedges.

Vegetable Gumbo

Yield: 6 cups (6 servings)
Serving Size: 1 cup gumbo
plus ½ cup rice
Exchanges:
Starch/Bread   2.0
Vegetable   2.0
Fat   0.5

Nutrient Content per Serving

CAL	235	*Na	59 (mg)
PRO	6 (gm)	K	473 (mg)
Fat	5.9 (gm)	Fiber	6 (gm)
CHO	42 (gm)	Chol	0 (mg)

*Add 133 mg if optional salt is used.

Ingredients

2 TABLESPOONS OLIVE OIL
2 TABLESPOONS FLOUR
1 14½-OUNCE CAN NO-SALT-ADDED TOMATOES
1 10½-OUNCE CAN REDUCED-SODIUM CHICKEN BROTH OR 1⅓ CUPS WATER
1 LARGE ONION, COARSELY CHOPPED (2 CUPS)
1 CUP SLICED CARROTS (5 OUNCES)
1 CUP SLICED CELERY (ABOUT 2 STALKS, 4 OUNCES)
2 CLOVES GARLIC, MINCED
1 BAY LEAF
1 TEASPOON DRIED THYME
¼ TEASPOON SALT (OPTIONAL)
¼ TEASPOON FRESHLY GROUND BLACK PEPPER
⅛ TEASPOON HOT PEPPER SAUCE
3 CUPS SLICED FRESH OR 10 OUNCES FROZEN SLICED OKRA, PARTIALLY THAWED TO SEPARATE

1 LARGE GREEN PEPPER, COARSELY CHOPPED (2 CUPS,
   8 OUNCES)
2 TEASPOONS FILÉ POWDER (OPTIONAL)
3 CUPS HOT COOKED BROWN RICE
½ CUP CHOPPED PARSLEY

Method

1. Heat oil in large saucepan or Dutch oven over medium heat. Add flour; cook and stir until a reddish-brown roux forms, about 5–6 minutes.
2. Gradually stir in tomatoes and broth or water; bring to a boil. Stir in onion, carrots, celery, garlic, bay leaf, thyme, salt (if desired), pepper, and pepper sauce. Reduce heat; cover and simmer 30 minutes or until carrots are almost tender.
3. Add okra, green pepper, and filé powder, if desired. Cover and simmer 15 minutes, stirring occasionally. Discard bay leaf. Serve over rice; sprinkle with parsley.

Method-Microwave

1. Combine oil and flour with a whisk in 2½-quart microwave-safe casserole. Cook uncovered on high power until a reddish-brown roux forms, about 6–8 minutes, whisking after each 2 minutes of cooking.
2. Stir in tomatoes, broth, onion, carrots, celery, garlic, bay leaf, thyme, salt (if desired), pepper, and pepper sauce. Cover and cook on high power until boiling, about 8 minutes. Reduce power to medium and cook 20–25 minutes, stirring twice.
3. Add okra, green pepper, and filé powder, if desired. Cover and cook at high power until boiling, about 3 minutes. Reduce power to medium and cook 8–10 minutes, stirring once. Discard bay leaf. Serve over rice; sprinkle with parsley.

Korean Noodle Salad

Yield: 6 cups (6 servings)
Serving Size: 1 cup

Exchanges: without cashews

Starch/Bread	2.0
Vegetable	1.0
Fat	1.0

with cashews

Starch/Bread	2.0
Vegetable	1.0
Fat	1.5

Nutrient Content per Serving

	without cashews	with cashews
CAL	224	242
PRO	6 (gm)	6 (gm)
Fat	8.2 (gm)	9.6 (gm)
CHO	33 (gm)	34 (gm)
Na	207 (mg)	208 (mg)
K	243 (mg)	260 (mg)
Fiber	3.1 (gm)	3.3 (gm)
Chol	0 (mg)	0 (mg)

Ingredients

- 8 OUNCES DRY CHINESE UDON NOODLES OR VERMI-CELLI, COOKED AND DRAINED
- 3 TABLESPOONS MILD ORIENTAL FLAVORED OIL (PAGE 143)
- 2 TABLESPOONS REDUCED-SODIUM SOY SAUCE
- 2 TABLESPOONS RICE WINE VINEGAR OR WHITE WINE VINEGAR
- ½ OUNCE DRIED SHIITAKE, PORCINI, OR TREE EAR MUSHROOMS, SOAKED, DRAINED, AND SLICED
- 4 OUNCES FRESH PEA PODS, BLANCHED AND CUT INTO THIN STRIPS
- 1 MEDIUM CARROT, SLICED WITH VEGETABLE PEELER INTO THIN STRIPS (2 OUNCES)
- 2 LARGE GREEN ONIONS WITH TOPS, DIAGONALLY CUT INTO ¼-INCH SLICES
- 1 CUP BEAN SPROUTS
- 2 TABLESPOONS CHOPPED DRY ROASTED UNSALTED CASHEWS (OPTIONAL)

Method

1. Toss hot cooked noodles with 1 tablespoon oil. Combine remaining oil with soy sauce and vinegar.

2. Combine noodles, mushrooms, pea pods, carrot, onions, and bean sprouts. Add oil mixture; toss well. Serve warm. Sprinkle with cashews, if desired.

Macaroni and Two-Cheese Casserole

Yield: 3 cups (4 servings)
Serving Size: ¾ cup
Exchanges:

		Nutrient Content per Serving		
		CAL	281	Na	293 (mg)
		PRO	13 (gm)	K	177 (mg)
Starch/Bread	2.5	Fat	9.9 (gm)	Fiber	1 (gm)
Meat, medium-fat	1.0	CHO	35 (gm)	Chol	13 (mg)
Fat	1.0				

Ingredients

- 4 OUNCES ELBOW, SMALL SHELL, OR ZITI MACARONI
- 2 TABLESPOONS MARGARINE, DIVIDED
- 2 TABLESPOONS FINELY CHOPPED SHALLOT OR ONION
- 1 TABLESPOON FLOUR
- 1 CUP SKIM MILK
- ½ CUP (2 OUNCES) SHREDDED SHARP REDUCED-FAT CHEDDAR CHEESE
- ½ CUP FRESH WHOLE WHEAT BREAD CRUMBS
- ¼ TEASPOON PAPRIKA, PREFERABLY HOT HUNGARIAN
- 2 TABLESPOONS FRESHLY GRATED PARMESAN OR ASIAGO CHEESE

Method

1. Cook macaroni according to package directions, omitting salt and fat. Drain well.
2. While macaroni is cooking, melt 1 tablespoon margarine in small saucepan over medium heat. Sauté shallot until tender, about 3 minutes. Add flour; cook and stir 1 minute. Add milk; cook until thickened, about 4 minutes, stirring occasionally.

(continued on page 262)

3. Stir in cheddar cheese until melted. Stir in macaroni. Transfer to gratin or shallow ovenproof baking dish.
4. Melt remaining margarine; combine with bread crumbs and Parmesan cheese. Sprinkle over macaroni.
5. Broil 4–5 inches from heat source until lightly browned, about 2 minutes.

Note: No need to give up traditional "comfort foods" now that they can be made lighter with new lower-fat products that are readily available.

Wild Rice–Stuffed Squash

Yield: 2 servings
Serving Size: ½ stuffed squash
Exchanges:
Starch/Bread   3.5
Fat   0.5

Nutrient Content per Serving

CAL	292	Na	124 (mg)
PRO	8 (gm)	K	741 (mg)
Fat	7.0 (gm)	Fiber	10.2 (gm)
CHO	52 (gm)	Chol	8 (mg)

Ingredients

1 MEDIUM ACORN SQUASH, ABOUT 1½ POUNDS, HALVED AND SEEDED
1 MEDIUM ONION, CUT INTO THIN WEDGES (6 OUNCES)
1 CLOVE GARLIC, MINCED
2 TEASPOONS MARGARINE
4 OUNCES SHIITAKE MUSHROOMS, STEMS DISCARDED, CAPS SLICED
1 TABLESPOON FRESH CHOPPED THYME LEAVES OR 1 TEASPOON DRIED THYME
1 CUP COOKED WILD OR BROWN RICE
¼ CUP (1 OUNCE) SHREDDED PART-SKIM OR SMOKED MOZZARELLA CHEESE

Method

1. Preheat oven to 375°F. Place squash cut side down in shallow baking dish. Bake 30 minutes.
2. While squash is baking, sauté onion and garlic in margarine in nonstick skillet until tender, about 4 minutes. Add mushrooms and thyme; cook and stir 3 minutes. Add rice; heat through.
3. Turn partially baked squash cut side up in same baking dish. Spoon rice mixture into squash halves; press down lightly and sprinkle with cheese.
4. Bake 15–20 minutes or until squash is tender.

Method-Microwave

1. Place squash cut side down in shallow microwave-safe baking dish. Cook uncovered on high power 10–12 minutes, rotating dish once. Remove and let stand while preparing stuffing.
2. Place margarine in same baking dish. Cook on high power until melted, about 45 seconds. Toss onion and garlic with margarine. Cover with vented plastic wrap. Cook on high power 3 minutes. Stir in mushrooms and thyme; cover and cook 3 minutes. Stir in rice.
3. Spoon into squash halves; press down lightly. Sprinkle with cheese. Wipe out baking dish; return stuffed squash to dish. Cover with waxed paper.
4. Cook on high power 5–7 minutes or until squash is tender. Let stand 5 minutes.

Note: To aid squash in standing upright in dish, cut small level slice off ends of cooked squash.

Two-Bean Chili

Yield: 7 cups (7 servings)
Serving Size: 1 cup
Exchanges:
Starch/Bread 2.0
Vegetable 1.0

Nutrient Content per Serving

CAL	174	*Na	210 (mg)
PRO	9 (gm)	K	669 (mg)
Fat	2.1 (gm)	Fiber	7.6 (gm)
CHO	32 (gm)	Chol	0 (mg)

*Add 76 mg if optional salt is used.

Ingredients

- 1 LARGE ONION, COARSELY CHOPPED (2 CUPS)
- 2 CLOVES GARLIC, MINCED
- 2 TEASPOONS OIL
- 1 14½-OUNCE CAN NO-SALT-ADDED STEWED TOMATOES
- 1 CAN OR BOTTLE BEER (12 OUNCES)
- 1 TABLESPOON CHILI POWDER
- 1 TEASPOON GROUND CUMIN
- 1 TEASPOON HOT PEPPER SAUCE OR HOT SALSA OR PICANTE SAUCE
- ¼ TEASPOON SALT (OPTIONAL)
- 1 15-OUNCE CAN PINTO BEANS, RINSED AND DRAINED
- 1 CAN (ABOUT 16 OUNCES) DARK RED KIDNEY BEANS, RINSED AND DRAINED
- 1 LARGE GREEN BELL PEPPER, COARSELY CHOPPED (2 CUPS, 8 OUNCES)
- ¼ CUP CHOPPED CILANTRO

Method

1. Sauté onion and garlic in large saucepan or Dutch oven in oil until tender, about 4 minutes. Stir in tomatoes, beer, chili powder, cumin, hot sauce, and salt, if desired.
2. Simmer uncovered 15 minutes. Stir in beans and green pepper. Simmer uncovered 15 minutes. Sprinkle with cilantro.

Method-Microwave

1. Toss onion and garlic with oil in 2½-quart microwave-safe casserole dish. Cover and cook on high power 3 minutes. Stir in tomatoes, beer, chili powder, cumin, hot sauce, and salt, if desired.
2. Cover and cook on high power until boiling, 5–6 minutes. Stir; reduce power to medium and cook 12 minutes, stirring once. Add beans and bell pepper.
3. Microwave version of chili will be thinner. If desired, combine 2 tablespoons cornstarch and 2 tablespoons water. Stir into chili; cover and cook on high power 2 minutes.

Note: Chili, soups, and stews freeze well in tightly covered plastic containers up to 6 months. Defrost and reheat in microwave oven for a quick lunch or dinner.

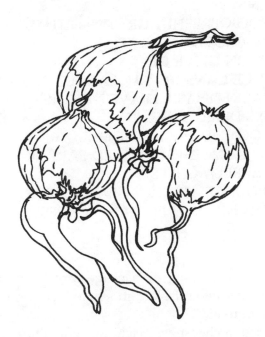

Spinach and Three-Cheese Lasagne

Yield: 8 servings
Serving Size: ⅛ recipe
Exchanges:
Starch/Bread   1.0
Meat, medium-fat   2.0
Vegetable   1.0

Nutrient Content per Serving

CAL	253	Na	307 (mg)
PRO	19 (gm)	K	657 (mg)
Fat	10.4 (gm)	Fiber	3 (gm)
CHO	23 (gm)	Chol	34 (mg)

Ingredients

- 4 OUNCES WHOLE WHEAT LASAGNE NOODLES
- 1 CONTAINER (ABOUT 15 OUNCES) PART-SKIM RICOTTA CHEESE
- 1 10-OUNCE PACKAGE FROZEN CHOPPED SPINACH, THAWED AND SQUEEZED DRY
- ¼ CUP EGG SUBSTITUTE OR 2 EGG WHITES, SLIGHTLY BEATEN
- ⅛ TEASPOON FRESHLY GRATED NUTMEG
- 2 GARLIC CLOVES, MINCED
- 1 TEASPOON OLIVE OIL
- 2 15-OUNCE CANS NO-SALT-ADDED TOMATO SAUCE
- ¼ CUP PACKED BASIL LEAVES, CHOPPED, OR 2 TEASPOONS DRIED BASIL
- 1 TEASPOON SUGAR (OPTIONAL)
- 2 CUPS (8 OUNCES) SHREDDED PART-SKIM MOZZARELLA CHEESE
- ¼ CUP (1 OUNCE) FRESHLY GRATED ASIAGO, ROMANO, OR PARMIGIANO-REGGIANO CHEESE

Method

1. Cook noodles according to package directions, omitting salt and fat. Drain well and place in single layer on waxed paper. Preheat oven to 350°F.
2. Combine ricotta cheese, spinach, egg substitute, and nutmeg; set aside.
3. Sauté garlic in oil 1 minute. Add tomato sauce, basil, and sugar, if desired. Simmer uncovered 10 minutes.

4. Spread ½ cup of the sauce evenly over 13-by-9-inch baking dish. Layer half of noodles over sauce. Spread with half of ricotta mixture; sprinkle with half of mozzarella cheese. Spoon half of sauce over all; repeat layering with remaining ingredients, ending with sauce.
5. Cover with foil; bake 30 minutes. Uncover and continue baking 15 minutes or until bubbly. Sprinkle with Asiago cheese; let stand 5–10 minutes before serving.

Method-Microwave

1. Prepare noodles and ricotta mixture as in steps 1 and 2 above.
2. Toss garlic with oil in 1½-quart microwave-safe dish. Cover and cook on high power 1 minute. Stir in tomato sauce, basil, and sugar, if desired. Cover and cook on high power until boiling, 5–6 minutes.
3. Build lasagne in 2-quart microwave-safe rectangular dish as in step 4 above.
4. Cover with vented plastic wrap and cook on medium power 20–25 minutes or until bubbly, rotating dish once. Sprinkle with Asiago cheese; let stand 5 minutes before serving.

Note: Whole wheat pasta and lasagne noodles can be found in health food stores or large supermarkets in the diet foods section. If unavailable, substitute regular lasagne noodles.

Summer Squash and Pasta Toss

Yield: 4 cups (4 servings)	Nutrient Content per Serving			
Serving Size: 2 cups	CAL	220	Na	163 (mg)
Exchanges:	PRO	7 (gm)	K	238 (mg)
Starch/Bread 1.0	Fat	10.3 (gm)	Fiber	2.4 (gm)
Vegetable 2.0	CHO	26 (gm)	Chol	13 (mg)
Fat 2.0				

Ingredients

> 4 OUNCES DRY SMALL PASTA SUCH AS ZITI,
> MOSTACCIOLI, BOW TIE, OR SMALL SHELLS (ABOUT
> 2 CUPS)
> 1 LARGE OR 2 MEDIUM ZUCCHINI SQUASH (8 OUNCES)
> 1 LARGE OR 2 MEDIUM YELLOW SQUASH (8 OUNCES)
> 2 TABLESPOONS EXTRA-VIRGIN OLIVE OIL
> 2 CLOVES GARLIC, MINCED
> ¼–½ TEASPOON RED PEPPER FLAKES
> ¼ CUP PACKED BASIL LEAVES, THINLY SLICED*
> ½ CUP (2 OUNCES) CRUMBLED FETA OR GOAT CHEESE
> FRESHLY GROUND BLACK PEPPER

Method

1. Cook pasta according to package directions, omitting salt and fat.
2. Slice squash ½ inch thick. Cut each slice in half or quarters, as desired. Add to boiling water with pasta during last 2 minutes of cooking.
3. Drain pasta and vegetables, reserving ¼ cup cooking liquid. Add oil, garlic, and pepper flakes to same pan. Cook over medium heat 2–3 minutes or until garlic is softened. Return drained pasta and vegetables to pan with reserved cooking liquid; toss well.
4. Stir in basil and cheese. Serve immediately with pepper.

*To substitute 1 teaspoon dried basil leaves, crushed, for fresh basil, add to oil with garlic.

Eggplant Parmesan

Yield: 4 servings	Nutrient Content per Serving			
Serving Size: ¼ recipe	CAL	101	Na	161 (mg)
Exchanges:	PRO	7 (gm)	K	456 (mg)
Meat, medium-fat 1.0	Fat	3.6 (gm)	Fiber	2.1 (gm)
Vegetable 2.0	CHO	12 (gm)	Chol	11 (mg)

Ingredients

1 MEDIUM EGGPLANT, UNPEELED AND SLICED INTO
½-INCH-THICK ROUNDS (1 POUND)
2 MEDIUM TOMATOES, SLICED
1 6-OUNCE CAN REDUCED-SODIUM COCKTAIL VEGE-
TABLE JUICE
2 TABLESPOONS CHOPPED FRESH BASIL OR 2
TEASPOONS DRIED BASIL
1 TEASPOON CHOPPED FRESH OREGANO LEAVES OR
¼ TEASPOON DRIED OREGANO
2 CLOVES GARLIC, MINCED
½ CUP (2 OUNCES) SHREDDED PART-SKIM
MOZZARELLA CHEESE
3 TABLESPOONS GRATED PARMESAN CHEESE

Method

1. Heat oven to 350°F. Layer eggplant and tomatoes into 8-inch
   square glass baking dish. Combine vegetable juice, basil, oregano, and garlic; pour over eggplant and tomatoes.
2. Cover with foil; bake 20 minutes. Uncover; sprinkle with
   mozzarella, then Parmesan cheese. Bake uncovered 15–20
   minutes or until golden brown.

Method-Microwave

1. Prepare casserole as directed in step 1 above.
2. Cover with vented plastic wrap. Cook on high power 7 minutes, rotating dish once. Uncover; sprinkle with mozzarella,
   then Parmesan cheese. Cover with waxed paper; cook on
   high power 5–7 minutes. Let stand 5 minutes before serving.

Thin Crust Spa Pizza

Yield: 4 servings
Serving Size: 1 pizza
Exchanges:

Starch/Bread	3.0
Meat, lean	1.0
Vegetable	2.0
Fat	1.0

Nutrient Content per Serving

CAL	393	Na	209 (mg)
PRO	20 (gm)	K	394 (mg)
Fat	11.3 (gm)	Fiber	5.4 (gm)
CHO	55 (gm)	Chol	24 (mg)

Ingredients

- ½ PACKAGE ACTIVE DRY QUICK-RISING YEAST (1½ TEASPOONS)
- 1 TEASPOON SUGAR
- ¾ CUP WARM WATER (110°–115°F)
- 1 CUP ALL-PURPOSE FLOUR
- 1 CUP WHOLE WHEAT FLOUR
- 1 TABLESPOON OLIVE OIL
  VEGETABLE COOKING SPRAY
- 1 TEASPOON CORNMEAL
- ½ CUP NO-SALT-ADDED TOMATO SAUCE
- 1 TABLESPOON CHOPPED FRESH BASIL LEAVES OR 1 TEASPOON DRIED BASIL
- 1½ CUPS SHREDDED PART-SKIM MOZZARELLA CHEESE (6 OUNCES)
- 1 RED BELL PEPPER, THINLY SLICED INTO RINGS (6 OUNCES)
- 4 THIN SLICES RED OR SWEET WHITE ONION, SEPARATED INTO RINGS (1 OUNCE)

Method

1. Stir yeast and sugar into water; let stand 5 minutes. Combine flours. Add yeast mixture and oil, stirring until dough forms. Knead by hand or in food processor fitted with plastic blade or mixer fitted with dough hook until smooth and elastic. Transfer to bowl that has been sprayed with nonstick cooking

spray and let rise in warm place until double in bulk, 20–30 minutes.

2. Heat oven to 450°F. Punch down dough. Transfer to lightly floured surface. Divide into 4 balls. Roll and stretch each portion of dough into circle, about 8 inches in diameter. Transfer to cookie sheet that has been sprayed with vegetable spray and sprinkled with cornmeal.

3. Combine tomato sauce and basil. Divide among 4 pizzas, spread evenly over dough, leaving a ½-inch border. Sprinkle each with 3 tablespoons cheese. Top with pepper and onion slices, then top with 3 tablespoons cheese.

4. Bake 10–12 minutes or until crust is golden brown and cheese is melted and bubbly.

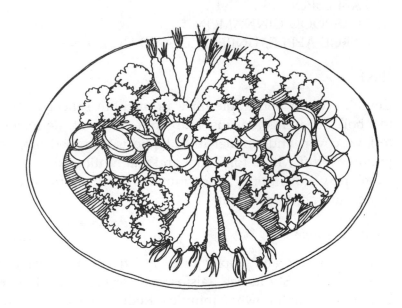

High-Fiber Fruit and Brown Rice Salad

Yield: 4 servings	Nutrient Content per Serving			
Serving Size: ¼ recipe	CAL	319	Na	162 (mg)
Exchanges:	PRO	5 (gm)	K	362 (mg)
Starch/Bread 2.5	Fat	2.5 (gm)	Fiber	5.9 (gm)
Fruit 2.0	CHO	72 (gm)	Chol	1 (mg)

Ingredients

    2 CUPS WATER
    ⅔ CUP UNSWEETENED APPLE JUICE OR CIDER
    1 CUP UNCOOKED BROWN RICE
    ⅓ CUP GOLDEN OR DARK RAISINS
    1 TEASPOON MARGARINE
    ¼ TEASPOON SALT
    ⅓ CUP PLAIN LOW-FAT YOGURT
    2 TABLESPOONS HONEY
    ½ TEASPOON CINNAMON
    1 LARGE APPLE, UNPEELED AND DICED

Method

1. Combine water and apple juice in medium saucepan. Bring to a boil. Stir in rice, raisins, margarine, and salt. Reduce heat to low, cover, and simmer until liquid is absorbed, about 50 minutes. Fluff with a fork; cool and chill until cold.
2. Combine yogurt, honey, and cinnamon in medium bowl. Stir in rice and apple; mix well.

Method-Microwave

1. Combine water and apple juice in 2-quart microwave-safe casserole dish. Stir in rice, raisins, margarine, and salt. Cover and cook on high power 5 minutes. Reduce power to medium and continue to cook 40–45 minutes or until most of liquid is absorbed, stirring twice. Let stand covered until all liquid is absorbed, about 5 minutes. Fluff with a fork; cool and chill until cold.
2. Continue as directed in step 2 above.

Ziti with Eggplant

Yield: 4 servings
Serving Size: ¼ recipe
Exchanges:
Starch/Bread   3.0
Vegetable   1.0
Fat   0.5

Nutrient Content per Serving

CAL	289	Na	178 (mg)
PRO	11 (gm)	K	199 (mg)
Fat	6.2 (gm)	Fiber	2.2 (gm)
CHO	47 (gm)	Chol	4 (mg)

Ingredients

  8 OUNCES ZITI OR MOSTACCIOLI PASTA, UNCOOKED
  ½ POUND JAPANESE OR REGULAR EGGPLANT,
    UNPEELED
  1 TABLESPOON OLIVE OIL
  2 CLOVES GARLIC, MINCED
  ¾ CUP REDUCED-SODIUM BEEF BROTH
  2 TABLESPOONS NO-SALT-ADDED TOMATO PASTE
  ¼ TEASPOON RED PEPPER FLAKES
  ¼ CUP PACKED BASIL LEAVES, SLICED THIN
  ¼ CUP (1 OUNCE) GRATED ASIAGO OR ROMANO
    CHEESE

Method

1. Cook pasta according to package directions, omitting salt and fat. While pasta is cooking, slice eggplant thinly (cut larger slices into pieces). Heat oil in large nonstick skillet. Sauté eggplant with garlic until lightly browned.
2. Add broth, tomato paste, and pepper flakes; cover and simmer uncovered 5 minutes or until pasta is ready.
3. Drain pasta; divide among 4 shallow bowls. Spoon eggplant and sauce over; sprinkle with basil and cheese.

Stir-Fried Vegetable Burritos

Yield: 8 burritos (4 servings)   Nutrient Content per Serving

Serving Size: 2 burritos		CAL	320	Na	313 (mg)
Exchanges:		PRO	8 (gm)	K	410 (mg)
Starch/Bread	3.0	Fat	8.6 (gm)	Fiber	5.8 (gm)
Vegetable	1.0	CHO	55 (gm)	Chol	0 (mg)
Fat	1.0				

Ingredients

    4 LARGE DRIED SHIITAKE MUSHROOMS
    1 TABLESPOON PEANUT OR VEGETABLE OIL
    2 CLOVES GARLIC, MINCED
    1 LARGE CARROT, CUT INTO JULIENNE STRIPS
    1 LARGE ZUCCHINI OR YELLOW SQUASH, CUT INTO
      JULIENNE STRIPS
    4 CUPS LOOSELY PACKED SLICED NAPA OR GREEN
      CABBAGE
    2 GREEN ONIONS, CUT INTO ½-INCH PIECES
  ¼ CUP REDUCED-SODIUM CHICKEN BROTH
    1 TABLESPOON REDUCED-SODIUM SOY SAUCE
    1 TEASPOON CORNSTARCH
    8 6-INCH-DIAMETER FLOUR TORTILLAS, HEATED
  ¼ CUP HOISIN SAUCE

Method

1. Discard stems from mushrooms. Soak caps in hot water to cover until soft. Squeeze dry and slice thinly.
2. Heat oil in wok or large skillet over medium-high heat. Add garlic, carrot, squash, and cabbage. Stir-fry until vegetables are crisp-tender, about 4 minutes. Stir in mushrooms and green onions.
3. Combine broth, soy sauce, and cornstarch; stir until smooth. Add to wok; cook and stir until thickened, about 1 minute.
4. Spread tortillas with hoisin sauce; divide vegetable mixture down center of each tortilla. Roll up; serve immediately.

Vegetable Tomato Sauce over Rigatoni

Yield: 6 servings
Serving Size: ⅙ recipe

Exchanges:

Starch/Bread	3.0
Vegetable	2.0
Fat	0.5

Nutrient Content per Serving

CAL	316	Na	138 (mg)
PRO	12 (gm)	K	722 (mg)
Fat	4.9 (gm)	Fiber	4.5 (gm)
CHO	58 (gm)	Chol	4 (mg)

Ingredients

- 1 LARGE ONION, CHOPPED
- 2 CLOVES GARLIC, MINCED
- 1 TABLESPOON OLIVE OIL
- 2 CUPS SLICED MUSHROOMS (ABOUT 4 OUNCES)
- 2 14½-OUNCE CANS NO-SALT-ADDED TOMATO SAUCE
- 1 CUP SHREDDED CARROTS
- ¼ CUP COARSELY CHOPPED FRESH BASIL LEAVES OR 1 TABLESPOON DRIED BASIL
- ½ TEASPOON RED PEPPER FLAKES
- 12 OUNCES UNCOOKED RIGATONI, COOKED WITHOUT SALT OR FAT, DRAINED
- ⅓ CUP FRESHLY GRATED ROMANO OR PARMESAN CHEESE

Method

1. Sauté onion and garlic in oil in large saucepan until tender, about 4 minutes. Add mushrooms; sauté 2 minutes.
2. Add tomato sauce, carrots, basil, and pepper flakes; simmer uncovered 20 minutes, stirring occasionally.
3. Serve over rigatoni; sprinkle with cheese.

Method-Microwave

1. Toss onion and garlic with oil in 2½- to 3-quart microwave-safe casserole. Cover and cook on high power 3 minutes. Add mushrooms; toss to coat. Cook uncovered on high power 4 minutes.

2. Add tomato sauce, carrots, basil, and pepper flakes; mix well. Cook uncovered on high power 10–12 minutes, stirring occasionally. Proceed as directed in step 3 above.

Baked Stuffed Onions with Spinach and Feta

Yield: 2 servings

Serving Size: 2 stuffed onion halves

Exchanges:

Starch/Bread	2.0
Vegetable	1.0
Fat	1.0

Nutrient Content per Serving

CAL	234	Na	361 (mg)
PRO	10 (gm)	K	761 (mg)
Fat	8.9 (gm)	Fiber	8.4 (gm)
CHO	33 (gm)	Chol	13 (mg)

Ingredients

2 VERY LARGE ONIONS (SPANISH OR SWEET WHITE WHEN IN SEASON), UNPEELED (ABOUT 1½ POUNDS)
2 TEASPOONS OLIVE OIL
1 CLOVE GARLIC, MINCED
1 10-OUNCE PACKAGE FROZEN CHOPPED SPINACH, DRAINED AND SQUEEZED DRY
1 TEASPOON LEMON JUICE
¼ TEASPOON FRESHLY GROUND BLACK PEPPER
¼ CUP DRY BREAD CRUMBS
¼ CUP (1 OUNCE) FETA CHEESE, CRUMBLED

Method

1. Boil onions in water to cover until partially tender, about 10–15 minutes. Cool; peel and cut in half crosswise. Scoop out center of onion, leaving ½-inch shell. Reserve centers. If necessary, cut small piece from ends of onions so they will stand upright. Place in shallow baking dish large enough to hold in one layer.

2. Heat oven to 350°F.
3. Chop centers of onion; sauté in oil with garlic in medium saucepan until tender, about 4 minutes. Stir in spinach, lemon juice, and pepper; cook until liquid is evaporated. Remove from heat; fold in bread crumbs and cheese.
4. Mound spinach mixture in onion shells. Cover with foil and bake until heated through, about 25 minutes.

Method-Microwave

1. Cut onions in half crosswise; peel and place cut side down in 9- or 10-inch microwave-safe pie plate. Cover with vented plastic wrap; cook on high power 6–8 minutes or until partially tender. Cool; scoop out center of onion, leaving ½-inch shell. Reserve centers. If necessary, cut small piece from ends of onions so they will stand upright. Return to pie plate; set aside.
2. Chop centers of onion; toss with garlic and oil in 1½-quart microwave-safe casserole. Cook uncovered at high power 2 minutes. Stir in spinach, lemon juice, and pepper. Cook uncovered at high power 3 minutes. Fold in bread crumbs and cheese.
3. Mound spinach mixture into onion shells. Cover with wax paper and cook on medium power 6–8 minutes or until heated through, rotating dish once. Let stand covered 5 minutes.

Side Dishes:
Grains, Potatoes,
Pasta

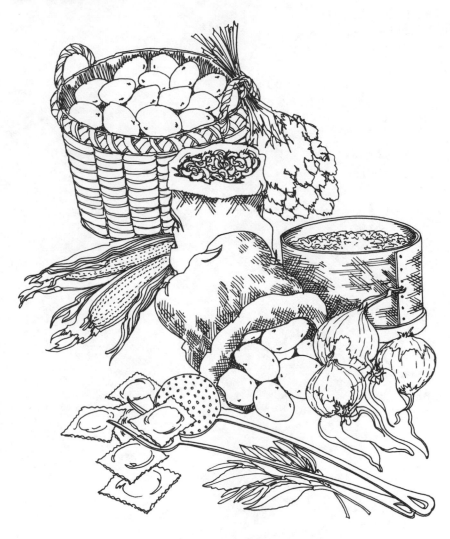

Sweet Potatoes with Lemon

Yield: 2 servings

Serving Size: 1 potato

Exchanges:

Starch/Bread 2.0

Fat 1.0

Nutrient Content per Serving

CAL	206	*Na	83 (mg)
PRO	3 (gm)	K	527 (mg)
Fat	5.8 (gm)	Fiber	3 (gm)
CHO	37 (gm)	Chol	0 (mg)

*Add 267 mg if optional salt is used.

Ingredients

    2 MEDIUM SWEET POTATOES (ABOUT 6 OUNCES EACH)
    1 TABLESPOON MARGARINE
    1 TABLESPOON FRESH LEMON JUICE
    ¼ TEASPOON SHREDDED LEMON PEEL
    ¼ TEASPOON SALT (OPTIONAL)
    ⅛ TEASPOON NUTMEG, PREFERABLY FRESHLY GRATED

Method

1. Scrub potatoes, pierce with tip of sharp knife in several places, and place in oven. Turn oven to 375°F. (Using a large toaster oven saves energy.)
2. Bake until potatoes are tender, about 45 minutes.
3. Slice open lengthwise with fork. Top with margarine. Sprinkle with lemon juice, peel, salt (if desired), and nutmeg. Serve immediately.

Method-Microwave

1. Scrub potatoes, pierce with tip of sharp knife in several places, and place on paper towel in oven.
2. Cook on high power 5–7 minutes or until tender, rotating once. Let stand 3 minutes.
3. Prepare potatoes as above in step 3.

Spanish Rice Picante

Yield: 1½ cups (2 servings) Nutrient Content per Serving
Serving Size: ¾ cup

Serving Size: ¾ cup	CAL	241	Na	207 (mg)
Exchanges:	PRO	6 (gm)	K	224 (mg)
Starch/Bread 3.0	Fat	3.4 (gm)	Fiber	2 (gm)
	CHO	46 (gm)	Chol	1 (mg)

Ingredients

½ CUP CHOPPED ONION
1 CLOVE GARLIC, MINCED
1 TEASPOON OLIVE OIL
½ CUP UNCOOKED CONVERTED RICE
1 CUP REDUCED-SODIUM CHICKEN BROTH
⅓ CUP PREPARED SALSA OR PICANTE SAUCE
½ CUP CHOPPED TOMATO
2 TABLESPOONS COARSELY CHOPPED CILANTRO

Method

1. Sauté onion and garlic in oil in small saucepan until tender, about 3 minutes.
2. Stir in rice; cook 1 minute. Add broth and salsa; bring to a boil.
3. Reduce to a simmer; cover and cook 20 minutes.
4. Stir in tomato; cover and let stand 5 minutes. Sprinkle with cilantro.

Method-Microwave

1. Toss onion and garlic with oil in 2-quart microwave-safe casserole. Cover and cook on high power 3 minutes. Stir in rice, broth, and salsa.
2. Cover and cook on high power until boiling, about 3–4 minutes.
3. Reduce power to medium and cook 18–20 minutes.
4. Stir in tomato; cover and let stand 5 minutes. Sprinkle with cilantro.

Note: Although rice cooked in the microwave oven does not save time, the advantage is that the rice can be prepared in a serving dish that makes cleanup easier. During hot summer months use your microwave oven as a much cooler cooking method.

Roasted Potatoes with Garlic and Rosemary

Yield: 2 servings
Serving Size: ½ potato

Nutrient Content per Serving

Exchanges:

		CAL	210	Na	331 (mg)
Starch/Bread	2.0	PRO	3 (gm)	K	574 (mg)
Fat	1.0	Fat	6.9 (gm)	Fiber	4 (gm)
		CHO	35 (gm)	Chol	0 (mg)

Ingredients

    1 LARGE BAKING POTATO
    1 TABLESPOON GARLIC-FLAVORED OLIVE OIL*
    ½ TEASPOON CRUSHED ROSEMARY
    ¼ TEASPOON SALT

Method:

1. Preheat oven to 350°F. Scrub potato; cut in half lengthwise. Cut each half lengthwise into 4 wedges.
2. Place in shallow baking dish. Combine oil, rosemary, and salt. Brush potatoes lightly with some of oil mixture.
3. Bake until tender and golden brown, about 1 hour, brushing with oil mixture every 15 minutes.

   *To make garlic-flavored olive oil, crush peeled garlic cloves slightly and heat in olive oil until very hot. Let stand 1 hour; discard garlic.

Note: The oil must be stored in the refrigerator to avoid bacterial growth. Oil may congeal, but will be pourable and will liquefy quickly.

Italian-Style Risotto with Dried Mushrooms

Yield: 2½ cups (5 servings)
Serving Size: ½ cup
Exchanges:
Starch/Bread   2.0

Nutrient Content per Serving

CAL	173	Na	92 (mg)
PRO	5 (gm)	K	122 (mg)
Fat	4.5 (gm)	Fiber	2 (gm)
CHO	28 (gm)	Chol	3 (mg)

Ingredients

  1¼ CUPS WATER
  1 CUP REDUCED-SODIUM CHICKEN BROTH
  ¼ CUP (¼ OUNCE) DRIED MUSHROOMS (CHINESE TREE
     EAR, PORCINI, MOREL, OR THE LIKE)
  1 LARGE ONION, FINELY CHOPPED
  1 CLOVE GARLIC, MINCED
  1 TABLESPOON OLIVE OIL
  ¾ CUP UNCOOKED ARBORIO RICE (ITALIAN SHORT-
     GRAINED)
  ¼ CUP DRY WHITE WINE
  ¼ CUP FRESHLY GRATED ASIAGO CHEESE

Method

1. Combine water, broth, and mushrooms in saucepan. Bring to a boil; reduce heat to simmer and simmer uncovered 10 minutes or until mushrooms are hydrated.
2. Remove mushrooms with slotted spoon; reserve. If mushrooms are large, chop coarsely. Keep broth mixture in saucepan at a bare simmer.
3. Heat oil in 10-inch skillet over medium heat. Sauté onion and garlic in oil until tender, about 5 minutes. Add rice; sauté 1 minute.
4. Add wine; sauté until absorbed. Add the broth mixture, ½ cup at a time, maintaining a simmer so that rice absorbs broth mixture slowly.
5. When rice has absorbed most of the broth mixture (about 25 minutes), stir in mushrooms and heat through. Continue to

add remaining broth mixture ¼ cup at a time until rice is creamy and slightly firm in the center.
6. Sprinkle with cheese and serve immediately.

Speedy Chive Potatoes

Yield: 1 cup (2 servings)	Nutrient Content per Serving		
Serving Size: ½ cup	CAL	68	Na	48 (mg)
Exchanges:	PRO	2 (gm)	K	190 (mg)
Starch/Bread 1.0	Fat	0.4 (gm)	Fiber	2 (gm)
	CHO	14 (gm)	Chol	1 (mg)

Ingredients

½ CUP WATER
¼ CUP LOW-FAT BUTTERMILK
⅔ CUP INSTANT MASHED POTATO FLAKES
1 TABLESPOON CHOPPED CHIVES OR GREEN ONION
    WITH TOP
⅛ TEASPOON FRESHLY GROUND BLACK PEPPER

Method

1. Bring water to a boil in small saucepan.
2. Stir in remaining ingredients; remove from heat.
3. Let stand covered 1 minute; stir with fork.

Method-Microwave

1. Place hot tap water in small microwave-safe bowl or serving dish.
2. Cook on high power until boiling, about 3 mnutes.
3. Stir in remaining ingredients; cook on high power 30 seconds. Cover and let stand 1 minute; stir with fork.

Cheese-Stuffed Potatoes

Yield: 4 servings
Serving Size: ½ stuffed potato
Exchanges:
Starch/Bread   2.0

Nutrient Content per Serving

CAL	148	Na	254 (mg)
PRO	7 (gm)	K	440 (mg)
Fat	2.6 (gm)	Fiber	2.9 (gm)
CHO	25 (gm)	Chol	10 (mg)

Ingredients

2 MEDIUM RUSSET BAKING POTATOES (ABOUT 1 POUND)
½ CUP (2 OUNCES) SHREDDED REDUCED-FAT CHEDDAR CHEESE
¼ CUP LOW-FAT BUTTERMILK OR SKIM MILK
¼ CUP FINELY CHOPPED GREEN ONION WITH TOP
¼ TEASPOON SALT
1 CLOVE GARLIC
⅛ TEASPOON FRESHLY GROUND BLACK PEPPER
HOT OR SWEET HUNGARIAN PAPRIKA (OPTIONAL)

Method

1. Heat oven to 400°F. Scrub potatoes; prick in several places with sharp knives. Bake until tender, about 50–60 minutes.
2. Slice potatoes in half lengthwise. Scoop out pulp, leaving ¼-inch shell.
3. Combine potato pulp, cheese, buttermilk, green onion, salt, garlic, and pepper. If desired, sprinkle with paprika.
4. Place in baking pan and bake 20 minutes or until heated through.

Method-Microwave

1. Scrub potatoes; prick in several places with sharp knife. Place on paper towel; cook on high power 9–10 minutes or until tender, turning potatoes over once.
2. Prepare potatoes as in steps 2 and 3 above.
3. Place in shallow microwave-safe dish and cook on high power 3–4 minutes or until heated through, rotating dish once.

Grits and Cheese Chili Pie

Yield: 8 servings

Serving Size: ⅛ wedge of pie

Exchanges:

Starch/Bread   1.0

Meat, medium-fat   0.5

Nutrient Content per Serving

CAL	110	Na	90 (mg)
PRO	6 (gm)	K	54 (mg)
Fat	3.2 (gm)	Fiber	1.8 (gm)
CHO	15 (gm)	Chol	10 (mg)

*Add 39 mg if whole egg is used.

Ingredients

    3 CUPS WATER
    ¾ CUP QUICK-COOKING HOMINY GRITS
    1 CUP (4 OUNCES) REDUCED-CHOLESTEROL MONTE-
      REY JACK CHEESE
    ⅓ CUP THINLY SLICED GREEN ONIONS WITH TOPS
    ¼ CUP EGG SUBSTITUTE OR 1 EGG, BEATEN
    ¼ TEASPOON HOT PEPPER SAUCE
    2 4-OUNCE CANS WHOLE GREEN CHILES, DRAINED
      AND PATTED DRY

Method

1. Preheat oven to 350°F.
2. Bring water to a boil in medium saucepan. Slowly stir in grits; simmer until thickened, about 3–5 minutes, stirring frequently.
3. Remove from heat; stir in cheese, onions, egg substitute, and pepper sauce.
4. Arrange chiles in 9-inch pie plate spoke fashion, with larger ends against edges of plate and tips toward center. Pour grits mixture evenly over chiles. Bake 30 minutes or until set. Let stand 5 minutes. Cut into wedges and serve warm.

Rice with Black-Eyed Peas

Yield: About 5 cups (6 servings)

Serving Size: about ¾ cup

Exchanges:

Starch/Bread   2.5

Nutrient Content per Serving

CAL	207	Na	104 (mg)
PRO	7 (gm)	K	215 (mg)
Fat	2.5 (gm)	Fiber	6 (gm)
CHO	39 (gm)	Chol	0 (mg)

Ingredients

    2 TEASPOONS OLIVE OIL
    1 CUP CHOPPED ONION
    2 CLOVES GARLIC, MINCED
    1 CUP UNCOOKED LONG-GRAIN RICE
    ½ TEASPOON RED PEPPER FLAKES
    2 CUPS REDUCED-SODIUM CHICKEN BROTH OR WATER
    ¼ CUP DRY WHITE WINE
    1 15-OUNCE CAN BLACK-EYED PEAS, RINSED AND
      DRAINED
    1 CUP CHOPPED FRESH TOMATO
    ¼ CUP COARSELY CHOPPED CILANTRO OR ITALIAN
      PARSLEY
      FRESHLY GROUND BLACK PEPPER

Method

1. Heat oil in large saucepan. Sauté onion and garlic 3 minutes. Stir in rice and pepper flakes; cook 1 minute.
2. Add broth and wine; bring to a boil. Reduce heat; cover and simmer 18 minutes. Stir in peas and tomato; heat through.
3. Remove from heat; stir in cilantro. Serve with pepper.

Method-Microwave

1. Toss onion and garlic in oil in 2½-quart microwave-safe casserole dish. Cover and cook on high power 2 minutes. Stir in rice and pepper flakes.
2. Add broth and wine; cover and cook until boiling, about 5 minutes. Reduce heat to medium power and continue to cook 17–18 minutes or until most of liquid is absorbed. Stir in

peas and tomato. Cover and cook on high power 1 minute.
3. Let stand covered 3 minutes. Stir in cilantro. Serve with pepper.

Note: This traditionally southern recipe for Hoppin' John is updated with wine and cilantro.

Potato Pancakes

Yield: 10 pancakes (5 servings)
Serving Size: 2 pancakes
Exchanges:
Starch/Bread   1.5
Fat   0.5

Nutrient Content per Serving

CAL	139	*Na	57 (mg)
PRO	3 (gm)	K	344 (mg)
Fat	3.2 (gm)	Fiber	2 (gm)
CHO	24 (gm)	**Chol	0 (mg)

*Add 213 mg if optional salt is used.
**Add 55 mg if whole egg is used.

Ingredients

2 LARGE BAKING POTATOES, PEELED AND COARSELY
  GRATED (ABOUT 1¼ POUNDS)
1 SMALL ONION, GRATED (3 OUNCES)
¼ CUP EGG SUBSTITUTE OR 1 EGG
¼ CUP FLOUR
½ TEASPOON SALT (OPTIONAL)
4 TEASPOONS MARGARINE

Method

1. Combine potatoes, onion, egg substitute, flour, and salt, if desired; mix well.
2. Heat a large nonstick skillet over medium heat. Melt 2 teaspoons margarine in skillet. Drop potato mixture by scant ¼ cupfuls into skillet; flatten with back of spatula.
3. Cook until browned, about 4–5 minutes per side. Keep warm in 225°F oven while cooking remaining potato mixture, adding remaining margarine as necessary. Serve immediately.

Apple Wild Rice

Yield: 2 cups (4 servings)
Serving Size: ½ cup
Exchanges:
Starch/Bread   1.0
Fruit   1.0

Nutrient Content per Serving

CAL	145	*Na	41 (mg)
PRO	4 (gm)	K	133 (mg)
Fat	2.6 (gm)	Fiber	2.7 (gm)
CHO	28 (gm)	Chol	0 (mg)

*Add 133 mg if optional salt is used.

Ingredients

½ CUP UNCOOKED WILD RICE
1 SMALL ONION, CUT INTO THIN WEDGES (3 OUNCES)
2 TEASPOONS MARGARINE
1 CUP UNSWEETENED APPLE JUICE
1 CUP REDUCED-SODIUM CHICKEN BROTH OR WATER
¼ TEASPOON SALT (OPTIONAL)
¼ TEASPOON CINNAMON
1 CUP DICED UNPEELED APPLE

Method

1. Wash rice in cold water and drain well. Sauté onion in margarine in medium saucepan until tender, about 4 minutes.
2. Add rice; cook and stir 1 minute. Add juice, broth, salt (if desired), and cinnamon. Bring to a boil; reduce heat. Cover and simmer until rice is tender and most of the liquid is absorbed, about 50 minutes.
3. Stir in apple; cover and let stand 5 minutes. Drain off any excess liquid before serving.

Method-Microwave

1. Wash rice in cold water and drain well. Place margarine in 2-quart microwave-safe casserole dish. Cook on high power until melted, about 30 seconds. Toss onion in margarine; cover and cook 2 minutes. Stir in rice.
2. Add juice, broth, salt (if desired), and cinnamon. Cover and cook on high power until boiling, 5–6 minutes. Reduce power

to medium and cook 40–45 minutes or until most of the liquid is absorbed.
3. Stir in apple; cover and let stand 5 minutes. Drain off any excess liquid before serving.

Golden Currant Pilaf with Cinnamon

Yield: 6 servings
Serving Size: ½ cup
Exchanges:
Starch/Bread   2.0

Nutrient Content per Serving

CAL	144	*Na	15 (mg)
PRO	3 (gm)	K	60 (mg)
Fat	2 (gm)	Fiber	1 (gm)
CHO	28 (gm)	Chol	0 (mg)

*Add 178 mg if optional salt is used.

Ingredients

    1 MEDIUM ONION, CHOPPED
    2 TEASPOONS PEANUT OR OLIVE OIL
    1 CUP UNCOOKED LONG-GRAIN RICE
    1 10½-OUNCE CAN REDUCED-SODIUM CHICKEN
      BROTH
    1 CUP WATER
    ½ CUP DRIED CURRANTS
    1 TEASPOON TURMERIC
    ½ TEASPOON CINNAMON
    ½ TEASPOON SALT (OPTIONAL)
    ¼ CUP CHOPPED PARSLEY

Method

1. Sauté onion in oil in medium saucepan until tender, about 4 minutes. Add rice; cook 1 minute. Stir in broth, water, currants, turmeric, cinnamon, and salt, if desired. Bring to a boil.
2. Reduce heat; cover and simmer until most of liquid is absorbed, about 18 minutes. Remove from heat; let stand covered 5 minutes. Stir in parsley.

(continued on page 292)

Method-Microwave

1. Toss onion in oil in 2-quart microwave-safe casserole dish. Cover and cook on high power 2–3 minutes. Stir in rice. Add broth, water, currants, turmeric, cinnamon, and salt, if desired. Cover and cook on high power until boiling, about 6 minutes.
2. Reduce power to medium and cook 16–18 minutes. Let stand covered 5 minutes. Stir in parsley.

Note: This is an Indian dish that is especially good with basmati rice, which may be found in specialty food stores or large supermarkets. It has a nutty flavor and rich aroma.

Creamy Polenta

Yield: 2 cups (4 servings)
Serving Size: ½ cup
Exchanges:
Starch/Bread   1.0
Fat   0.5

Nutrient Content per Serving

CAL	103	Na	121 (mg)
PRO	5 (gm)	K	60 (mg)
Fat	2.5 (gm)	Fiber	1.6 (gm)
CHO	15 (gm)	Chol	3 (mg)

Ingredients

> 2 CUPS REDUCED-SODIUM CHICKEN BROTH OR
>   HOMEMADE (PAGE 118)
> ½ CUP YELLOW OR WHITE CORNMEAL
> ¼ CUP FRESHLY GRATED PARMESAN CHEESE

Method

1. Combine broth and cornmeal in medium saucepan. Bring to a boil, stirring frequently. Reduce heat and simmer over low heat until thickened, but creamy, about 12–15 minutes. Stir often to prevent sticking.
2. Remove from heat. Sprinkle with cheese.

Method-Microwave

1. Combine broth and cornmeal in 2-quart microwave-safe bowl. Cook uncovered on high power 7–9 minutes, or until thickened but creamy, stirring each 2 minutes.
2. Sprinkle with cheese.

Note: Polenta makes a good base for a meatless main dish. Top with a favorite tomato or mushroom sauce. It will keep warm covered 10 minutes before serving. Leftovers may be refrigerated, sliced, and sautéed in a small amount of olive oil in a nonstick pan for a second meal.

New Potatoes with Olive Oil and Garlic

Yield: 2 servings
Serving Size: ½ recipe
Exchanges:
Starch/Bread 2.0
Fat 1.0

Nutrient Content per Serving

CAL	207	*Na	8 (mg)
PRO	3 (gm)	K	564 (mg)
Fat	6.9 (gm)	Fiber	3.4 (gm)
CHO	34 (gm)	Chol	0 (mg)

*Add 267 mg if optional salt is used.

Ingredients

    12 OUNCES NEW (RED BOILING) POTATOES (ABOUT
        6–8 SMALL)
    1 TABLESPOON EXTRA-VIRGIN OLIVE OIL
    1 CLOVE GARLIC, MINCED
    ¼ TEASPOON SALT (OPTIONAL)
    FRESHLY GROUND BLACK PEPPER

Method

1. Peel off ½-inch strip of skin around center of each potato.
2. Place in steamer set over simmering water. Cover and steam until tender, 15–20 minutes.
3. Drain and reserve potatoes. Add oil and garlic to pan. Cook over medium heat until garlic is fragrant, about 2 minutes. Add potatoes and salt, if desired. Toss well. Serve with pepper.

Method-Microwave

1. Peel off ½-inch strip of skin around center of each potato.
2. Place potatoes in shallow microwave-safe dish. Add ½ cup water. Cover and cook on high power 4 minutes. Reduce power to medium and cook until potatoes are tender, 9–11 minutes.
3. Drain and reserve potatoes. Add oil and garlic to dish. Cook uncovered at high power 1–2 minutes or until garlic is fragrant. Add potatoes and salt, if desired. Toss well. Serve with pepper.

Vermont-Style Sweet Potatoes

Yield: 2 cups (4 servings)	Nutrient Content per Serving	
Serving Size: ½ cup	CAL 130	Na 43 (mg)
Exchanges:	PRO 2 (gm)	K 320 (mg)
Starch/Bread 1.5	Fat 2.9 (gm)	Fiber 2.1 (gm)
	CHO 25 (gm)	Chol 0 (mg)

Ingredients

> 2 LARGE SWEET POTATOES, PEELED AND QUARTERED
> (1 POUND)
> 1 TABLESPOON MARGARINE
> 1 TABLESPOON PURE MAPLE SYRUP
> 2 TEASPOONS FINELY GRATED ORANGE PEEL
> ⅛ TEASPOON FRESHLY GRATED NUTMEG

Method

1. Place potatoes in saucepan large enough to hold in one layer. Add water to cover. Bring to a boil; reduce heat. Cover and simmer until tender, about 15 minutes.
2. Drain, reserving 2 tablespoons of the water. Using potato masher, mash potatoes with margarine, syrup, orange peel, and nutmeg. Or transfer all ingredients to food processor fitted with steel blade and process with quick on/off turns just until potatoes are mashed. Do not overprocess or potatoes will become pasty.

Method-Microwave

1. Place potatoes in microwave-safe dish large enough to hold potatoes in one layer. Add 1 cup hot tap water. Cover with vented plastic wrap. Cook on high power until potatoes are tender, 10–12 minutes, rotating dish once.
2. Proceed as directed above in step 2.

Spicy Black Beans

Yield: 4 servings
Serving Size: ½ cup
Exchanges:
Starch/Bread 1.0
Vegetable 1.0
Fat 0.5

Nutrient Content per Serving

CAL	138	Na	225 (mg)
PRO	8 (gm)	K	407 (mg)
Fat	2.7 (gm)	Fiber	5.3 (gm)
CHO	22 (gm)	Chol	0 (mg)

Ingredients

    2 TEASPOONS OLIVE OIL
    1 CLOVE GARLIC, MINCED
    1 16-OUNCE CAN BLACK BEANS, RINSED AND DRAINED
    ⅓ CUP PREPARED SALSA OR PICANTE SAUCE
    1 TABLESPOON LIME JUICE
    1 MEDIUM TOMATO, SEEDED AND CHOPPED
    ¼ CUP COARSELY CHOPPED CILANTRO

Method

1. Heat oil in medium saucepan. Sauté garlic until tender, about 2 minutes. Add beans, salsa, and lime juice. Simmer until heated through, about 5 minutes, stirring occasionally.
2. Stir in tomato; sprinkle with cilantro.

Method-Microwave

1. Combine oil and garlic in 1½-quart microwave-safe casserole dish. Cook uncovered on high power 1 minute. Add beans, salsa, and lime juice. Cover and cook on high power 4–6 minutes, or until heated through, stirring once.
2. Stir in tomato; sprinkle with cilantro.

Pasta with Scallions and Garlic

Yield: 4 servings
Serving Size: ¼ recipe
Exchanges:
Starch/Bread   1.5
Fat   1.0

Nutrient Content per Serving

CAL	164	*Na	17 (mg)
PRO	4 (gm)	K	99 (mg)
Fat	7.1 (gm)	Fiber	3.8 (gm)
CHO	23 (gm)	Chol	0 (mg)

*Add 267 mg if optional salt is used.

Ingredients

    4 OUNCES WHOLE WHEAT SPAGHETTI
    2 TABLESPOONS GOOD-QUALITY OLIVE OIL
    2 CLOVES GARLIC, MINCED
    ½ CUP (ABOUT 3) DIAGONALLY SLICED GREEN ON-
    IONS WITH TOPS
    ½ TEASPOON FINELY SHREDDED LEMON PEEL
    ½ TEASPOON SALT (OPTIONAL)
    FRESHLY GROUND BLACK PEPPER

Method

1. Cook spaghetti in large saucepan according to package directions, omitting fat and salt.
2. Drain spaghetti in colander. Add oil to saucepan; sauté garlic in oil until tender, about 3 minutes. Return drained spaghetti to saucepan; toss to coat.
3. Add scallions, lemon peel and salt, if desired. Toss well until heated through. Sprinkle with pepper and serve immediately.

Great Plains Side Dish Stuffing

Yield: 4 cups
Serving Size: ½ cup
Exchanges:
Starch/Bread   1.0
Fat   0.5

Nutrient Content per Serving

CAL	97	*Na	107 (mg)
PRO	2 (gm)	K	95 (mg)
Fat	5.1 (gm)	Fiber	1.7 (gm)
CHO	11 (gm)	Chol	0 (mg)

*Add 67 mg if optional salt is used.

Ingredients

- 4 CUPS DAY-OLD FRENCH, SOURDOUGH, OR ITALIAN BREAD CUT IN ¾-INCH CUBES
- 2 TABLESPOONS MARGARINE
- 2 TABLESPOON OLIVE OIL
- 1 LARGE ONION, CHOPPED
- 1 LARGE RED BELL PEPPER, CHOPPED
- ½ CUP FROZEN CORN KERNELS, THAWED
- 1 TABLESPOON WATER (OR MORE IF MOISTER STUFFING IS DESIRED)
- ¼ CUP CHOPPED PARSLEY
- ¼ CUP SLICED GREEN ONIONS
- ¼ TEASPOON SALT (OPTIONAL)
- ¼ TEASPOON FRESHLY GROUND BLACK PEPPER

Method

1. Heat oven to 275°F.
2. Place bread cubes in single layer on baking sheet. Bake 20 minutes or until crisp and dry. Increase oven temperature to 350°F.
3. Melt margarine with oil in large saucepan. Sauté onion 2 minutes; add bell pepper and corn. Sauté 2 minutes. Add remaining ingredients, including bread cubes; toss well.
4. Transfer to medium baking dish. Cover and bake at 350°F until heated through, about 30–35 minutes.

Method-Microwave

1. Prepare bread cubes as in steps 1 and 2 above.
2. Combine margarine and oil in 3-quart microwave-safe casserole. Cook on high power until margarine is melted, about 45 seconds. Toss onion with margarine mixture. Cover and cook on high power 3 minutes. Add bell pepper and corn; cover and cook on high power 2 minutes. Stir in remaining ingredients, including bread cubes; toss well.
3. Cover with waxed paper; cook at high power until heated through, about 6–8 minutes. Let stand 5 minutes.

Vegetables

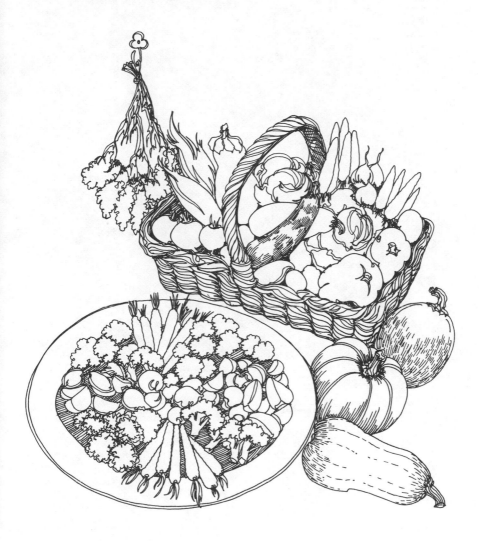

Asparagus with Dijon Sauce

Yield: 4 servings

Serving Size: ¼ recipe

Exchanges:

Vegetable   1.0

Nutrient Content per Serving

CAL	20	Na	60 (mg)
PRO	2 (gm)	K	120 (mg)
Fat	0.7 (gm)	Fiber	1 (gm)
CHO	2 (gm)	Chol	1 (mg)

Ingredients

    ¾ POUND FRESH ASPARAGUS SPEARS
    ¼ CUP REDUCED-SODIUM CHICKEN BROTH
    2 TEASPOONS DIJON MUSTARD OR TARRAGON DIJON
      MUSTARD
    1 TABLESPOON GRATED ROMANO OR ASIAGO CHEESE

Method

1. Break woody ends off asparagus; place in skillet.
2. Pour broth over; cover and steam over medium heat until crisp-tender, about 4 minutes.
3. Remove asparagus to warm serving plate with slotted spatula; keep warm.
4. Add mustard to skillet; increase heat to high and bring to a boil, stirring constantly.
5. Pour over asparagus; sprinkle with cheese.

Method-Microwave

1. Break woody ends off asparagus; place in 2-quart rectangular microwave-safe dish.
2. Pour broth over; cover with vented plastic wrap and cook on high power 3–4 minutes or until crisp-tender.
3. Pour off liquid into 1-cup glass measure. Keep asparagus covered.
4. Whisk mustard into juices. Cook uncovered at high power until boiling, about 30 seconds.
5. Pour over asparagus; sprinkle with cheese.

Broiled Tomatoes Parmesan

Yield: 4 servings
Serving Size: ½ tomato
Exchanges:
Vegetable 1.0
Fat 0.5

Nutrient Content per Serving

CAL	58	Na	59 (mg)
PRO	2 (gm)	K	187 (mg)
Fat	3 (gm)	Fiber	1 (gm)
CHO	7 (gm)	Chol	1 (mg)

Ingredients

2 RIPE MEDIUM TOMATOES (12–14 OUNCES)
1 CLOVE GARLIC, MINCED
2 TEASPOONS OLIVE OIL
1 TABLESPOON MINCED FRESH BASIL OR 1 TEASPOON DRIED BASIL
¼ TEASPOON FRESHLY GROUND BLACK PEPPER
½ CUP FRESH BREAD CRUMBS
1 TABLESPOON FRESHLY GRATED PARMESAN CHEESE (PREFERABLY IMPORTED PARMIGIANO-REGGIANO)

Method

1. Cut tomatoes in half crosswise. Squeeze out seeds and discard. Place cut side up on broiler pan.
2. Combine garlic, oil, basil, and pepper. Spread evenly over cut surfaces of tomatoes. Broil 6 inches from heat source until hot, about 5 minutes.
3. Combine crumbs and cheese; sprinkle evenly over hot tomatoes. Return to broiler until crumbs are browned, about 2 minutes. Serve immediately.

Braised Garlic

Yield: ½ cup cooked, peeled cloves (about 25 medium) (4 servings)
Serving Size: About 6 cloves or 2 tablespoons
Exchanges:
Vegetable   1.0

Nutrient Content per Serving

CAL	25	Na	6 (mg)
PRO	1 (gm)	K	75 (mg)
Fat	0 (gm)	Fiber	0 (gm)
CHO	6 (gm)	Chol	0 (mg)

Ingredients

    2 WHOLE HEADS GARLIC, SEPARATED INTO CLOVES
        BUT NOT PEELED
    ¼ CUP REDUCED-SODIUM CHICKEN BROTH
    2 TEASPOONS OLIVE OIL

Method

1. Combine garlic, broth, and oil in small saucepan.
2. Cover and simmer over low heat until garlic is tender, about 15 minutes.
3. Drain off liquid and discard. Press garlic out of skin. Use as a spread in place of butter or serve with chicken or pork.

Method-Microwave

1. Combine garlic, broth, and oil in small microwave-safe dish.
2. Cover tightly and cook on high power 2 minutes. Reduce power to medium and continue cooking 5–6 minutes. Let stand 20 minutes.
3. Drain off liquid and discard. Press garlic out of skin. Use as a spread in place of butter or serve with chicken or pork.

Three-Minute Pea Pods

Yield: 2 servings

Serving Size: ½ recipe

Exchanges:

Vegetable 2.0

Fat 0.5

Nutrient Content per Serving

CAL	80	Na	5 (mg)
PRO	3 (gm)	K	224 (mg)
Fat	2.8 (gm)	Fiber	3 (gm)
CHO	11 (gm)	Chol	0 (mg)

Ingredients

    1 TEASPOON SAFFLOWER OIL
    6 OUNCES FRESH PEA PODS OR FROZEN (UNTHAWED)
    ½ CUP SHORT, THIN RED OR YELLOW BELL PEPPER
        STRIPS (1½ OUNCES)
    1 CLOVE GARLIC, MINCED
    2 TEASPOONS ORANGE MARMALADE OR CONSERVE
    1 TEASPOON SHREDDED FRESH GINGERROOT

Method

1. Heat oil in wok or large skillet over medium-high heat.
2. Stir-fry pea pods, pepper, and garlic until crisp-tender about 3 minutes. Add marmalade and ginger; toss to coat.

Method-Microwave

1. Toss pea pods, pepper, and garlic with oil in 1-quart microwave-safe dish. Cook on high power 2–3 minutes or until crisp-tender.
2. Add marmalade and ginger; toss to coat.

Sugar Snap Peas with Basil and Lemon

Yield: 2 servings	Nutrient Content per Serving			
Serving Size: ½ recipe	CAL	89	Na	136 (mg)
Exchanges:	PRO	3 (gm)	K	276 (mg)
Vegetable 2.0	Fat	2.2 (gm)	Fiber	6 (gm)
Fat 0.5	CHO	14 (gm)	Chol	0 (mg)

Ingredients

1 TEASPOON OLIVE OIL
¾ POUND SUGAR SNAP PEAS OR 1 10-OUNCE PACK-
    AGE FROZEN SUGAR SNAP PEAS, THAWED (DO
    NOT THAW IF PREPARING IN MICROWAVE)
¼ TEASPOON SALT
¼ TEASPOON GROUND WHITE PEPPER
¼ CUP COARSELY CHOPPED FRESH BASIL LEAVES
½ TEASPOON GRATED LEMON PEEL
    LEMON WEDGES

Method

1. Heat oil in wok or nonstick skillet over medium heat.
2. Sprinkle peas with salt and pepper. Stir-fry peas until crisp-tender, 3 minutes for fresh or 2 minutes for frozen.
3. Add basil and lemon peel; stir-fry until basil is wilted and fragrant. Serve immediately with lemon wedges.

Method-Microwave

1. Sprinkle frozen or fresh peas with salt and pepper; toss with oil in 1-quart microwave-safe dish.
2. Cover and cook on high power 2–3 minutes for fresh or 1–2 minutes for frozen or until crisp-tender.
3. Stir in basil and lemon peel; cover and cook on high 1 minute. Serve with lemon wedges.

New England Red Cabbage

Yield: 4 cups (6 servings)	Nutrient Content per Serving			
Serving Size: ¾ cup	CAL	62	Na	100 (mg)
Exchanges:	PRO	1 (gm)	K	217 (mg)
Vegetable 2.0	Fat	1.7 (gm)	Fiber	3 (gm)
	CHO	12 (gm)	Chol	0 (mg)

Ingredients

- 1 CUP COARSELY CHOPPED ONION
- 2 TEASPOONS OLIVE OIL
- 1 SMALL RED CABBAGE (1 POUND), COARSELY CHOPPED (6 CUPS)
- ¼ CUP UNSWEETENED APPLE JUICE
- 2 TABLESPOONS RED WINE VINEGAR
- 2 TABLESPOONS BROWN SUGAR
- ½ TEASPOON GROUND CORIANDER
- ¼ TEASPOON SALT
- ¼ TEASPOON FRESHLY GROUND BLACK PEPPER
- ⅛ TEASPOON GROUND CINNAMON

Method

1. Sauté onion in oil in 10-inch skillet over medium heat 3 minutes. Stir in remaining ingredients; bring to a boil.
2. Reduce heat; cover and simmer 25 minutes, stirring occasionally.

Mushrooms in Creamy Sauce

Yield: 1 cup (2 servings)   Nutrient Content per Serving
Serving Size: ½ cup   CAL   65   Na   51 (mg)
Exchanges: PRO   3 (gm)   K   284 (mg)
Vegetable   1.0   Fat   3.9 (gm) Fiber   3 (gm)
Fat   1.0   CHO   5 (gm)   Chol   13 (mg)

Ingredients

    NONSTICK VEGETABLE SPRAY
  8 OUNCES SMALL MUSHROOMS, STEMS TRIMMED
  1 CLOVE GARLIC, MINCED
  1 TEASPOON BALSAMIC VINEGAR
  ¼ TEASPOON FRESHLY GROUND BLACK PEPPER
  ⅛ TEASPOON SALT
  1 OUNCE REDUCED-FAT CREAM CHEESE
    (NEUFCHÂTEL), CUBED
  2 TABLESPOONS THINLY SLICED GREEN ONIONS WITH
    TOPS

Method

1. Spray nonstick skillet with vegetable spray.
2. Cook mushrooms and garlic in skillet over medium heat 3 minutes, stirring constantly.
3. Add vinegar, pepper, and salt; cook and stir 1 minute.
4. Add cream cheese and green onions; cook and stir until melted and bubbly, about 2 minutes.

Method-Microwave

1. Combine mushrooms and garlic in shallow microwave-safe dish.
2. Cover and cook on high power 3–4 minutes, stirring once.
3. Add vinegar, pepper, and salt; cover and cook 1 minute.
4. Add cream cheese and green onions; cook 1–2 minutes. Stir; let stand covered 2 minutes.

Spinach with Bacon and Mushrooms

Yield: 1½ cups (2 servings) Nutrient Content per Serving

Serving Size: ¾ cup		CAL	101	Na	145 (mg)
Exchanges:		PRO	5 (gm)	K	709 (mg)
Vegetable	1.0	Fat	7.1 (gm)	Fiber	4 (gm)
Fat	1.5	CHO	7 (gm)	Chol	8 (mg)

Ingredients

　　1 SLICE BACON, DICED
　　¼ CUP FINELY CHOPPED ONION
　　1½ CUPS SLICED MUSHROOMS (4 OUNCES)
　　8 OUNCES FRESH SPINACH LEAVES, STEMS REMOVED
　　　FRESHLY GROUND BLACK PEPPER

Method

1. Cook bacon in 10-inch nonstick skillet over medium heat until crisp. Remove with slotted spoon to paper towel; reserve.
2. Cook onion in drippings 1 minute. Add mushrooms; cook and stir until tender, about 4 minutes.
3. Add spinach; cook and stir until wilted, about 1 minute. Sprinkle with reserved bacon. Serve with pepper.

Method-Microwave

1. Place bacon in shallow 2-quart microwave-safe dish. Cook uncovered on high power 2–3 minutes or until crisp.
2. Toss onion and mushrooms in drippings; cover and cook on high power 4–5 minutes, stirring once.
3. Stir in spinach; cover and cook on high power 2 minutes. Stir and sprinkle with reserved bacon. Serve with pepper.

Sweet Pepper and Onion Sauté

Yield: 2 cups (4 servings)
Serving Size: ½ cup
Exchanges:
Vegetable   1.0
Fat   0.5

Nutrient Content per Serving

CAL	54	Na	135 (mg)
PRO	1 (gm)	K	157 (mg)
Fat	3.7 (gm)	Fiber	2 (gm)
CHO	5 (gm)	Chol	0 (mg)

Ingredients

- 1 SMALL YELLOW BELL PEPPER (5 OUNCES)
- 1 SMALL RED BELL PEPPER (5 OUNCES)
- 1 SMALL GREEN, ORANGE, OR PURPLE BELL PEPPER (5 OUNCES)
- 1 TABLESPOON EXTRA-VIRGIN OLIVE OIL
- 1 MEDIUM ONION, CUT INTO THIN WEDGES
- 1 CLOVE GARLIC, MINCED
- ⅛ TEASPOON SALT

Method

1. Cut peppers lengthwise into thin strips.
2. Heat oil in large nonstick skillet over medium-high heat until very hot. Add peppers and onion; stir-fry 3 minutes.
3. Add garlic; continue to stir-fry 2–3 minutes or until tender. Sprinkle with salt.

Method-Microwave

1. Cut peppers lengthwise into thin strips.
2. Toss peppers, onion, and garlic with oil in 2-quart microwave-safe dish.
3. Cover and cook on high power 6–7 minutes or until tender, stirring once. Sprinkle with salt.

Spicy Corn Relish

Yield: 2 cups (4 servings)
Serving Size: ½ cup
Exchanges:
Vegetable 2.0
Fat 0.5

Nutrient Content per Serving

CAL	74	*Na	56 (mg)
PRO	2 (gm)	K	177 (mg)
Fat	2.6 (gm)	Fiber	3 (gm)
CHO	13 (gm)	Chol	0 (mg)

*Add 67 mg if optional salt is used.

Ingredients

> 2 TEASPOONS OLIVE OIL
> 1 CUP CHOPPED ONION
> 1 CLOVE GARLIC, MINCED
> 1 CUP FRESH OR FROZEN CORN KERNELS
> ½ CUP DICED RED BELL PEPPER
> ½ CUP DICED GREEN BELL PEPPER
> 1–2 TABLESPOONS FINELY CHOPPED PICKLED
>   JALAPEÑO PEPPERS
> ⅛ TEASPOON SALT (OPTIONAL)

Method

1. Heat oil in nonstick skillet. Add onion and garlic; sauté until tender, about 4 minutes.
2. Add corn, diced peppers, and jalapeño pepper. Sauté until diced peppers are crisp-tender, about 3 minutes.
3. Sprinkle with salt, if desired. Serve warm or chill and serve as salad or accompaniment to grilled meat or poultry.

Method-Microwave

1. Toss onion and garlic with oil in shallow microwave-safe dish. Cover and cook on high power 3 minutes.
2. Stir in diced peppers and jalapeño pepper. Cover and cook on high power 3–4 minutes or until diced peppers are crisp-tender.
3. Serve as directed above.

Mushroom-Dill Sauté

Yield: 2 cups (4 servings)
Serving Size: ½ cup
Exchanges:

		Nutrient Content per Serving			
		CAL	46	Na	67 (mg)
		PRO	1 (gm)	K	213 (mg)
Vegetable	1.0	Fat	3.2 (gm)	Fiber	2 (gm)
Fat	0.5	CHO	4 (gm)	Chol	0 (mg)

Ingredients

   1 TABLESPOON MARGARINE
   8 OUNCES MUSHROOMS, SLICED
   1 CUP YELLOW OR RED BELL PEPPER STRIPS (3 OUNCES)
   1 CLOVE GARLIC, MINCED
   2 TEASPOONS DIJON MUSTARD
   ¼ CUP CHOPPED FRESH DILL OR 1½ TEASPOONS DRIED
   DILL WEED
   FRESHLY GROUND BLACK PEPPER

Method

1. Melt margarine in 10-inch skillet over medium heat.
2. Sauté mushrooms, pepper strips, and garlic until mushrooms are tender and liquid is evaporated, about 5 minutes.
3. Stir in mustard; toss to coat. Stir in dill; heat through. Serve with pepper.

Method-Microwave

1. Place margarine in shallow 2-quart microwave-safe dish. Cook on high power until melted, about 45 seconds.
2. Toss mushrooms, pepper strips, and garlic with margarine. Cover and cook on high power 4–5 minutes, stirring once. Drain off excess liquid.
3. Stir in mustard until coated. Stir in dill. Cover and cook on high power 1 minute. Serve with pepper.

Grilled Red Onions

Yield: 4 servings
Serving Size: ½ grilled red onion
Exchanges:
Vegetable 1.0
Fat 1.0

Nutrient Content per Serving

CAL	88	*Na	2 (mg)
PRO	1 (gm)	K	133 (mg)
Fat	6.9 (gm)	Fiber	2.5 (gm)
CHO	6 (gm)	Chol	0 (mg)

*Add 67 mg if salt was used in Balsamic Vinaigrette.

Ingredients

2 MEDIUM RED ONIONS
¼ CUP BALSAMIC VINAIGRETTE (PAGE 129)
FRESHLY GROUND BLACK PEPPER

Method

1. Peel onions, leaving root end intact. Cut each onion into ½-inch wedges. Place in shallow dish or pie plate.
2. Drizzle with vinaigrette. Let stand at room temperature 30 minutes while preparing charcoal grill. Thread onion wedges onto skewers. Reserve vinaigrette.
3. Place on rack over medium coals or on broiler pan 4–5 inches from heat source. Grill or broil until tender, about 5 minutes per side, basting with vinaigrette. Serve with pepper.

Steamed Artichoke with Herbed Mustard Sauce

Yield: 2 servings
Serving Size: ½ large artichoke plus 1 tablespoon sauce
Exchanges:
Vegetable 1.0
Fat 1.5

Nutrient Content per Serving

CAL	94	Na	107 (mg)
PRO	2 (gm)	K	183 (mg)
Fat	7.1 (gm)	Fiber	2.6 (gm)
CHO	7 (gm)	Chol	0 (mg)

Ingredients

1 LARGE ARTICHOKE (¾ POUND)
1 CUP WATER
2 TEASPOONS BLACK PEPPERCORNS
1 TEASPOON FENNEL SEEDS
1 TABLESPOON PLUS 1 TEASPOON LEMON JUICE
1 TABLESPOON EXTRA-VIRGIN OLIVE OIL
2 TEASPOON DIJON-STYLE MUSTARD WITH
TARRAGON OR REGULAR DIJON MUSTARD PLUS ½
TEASPOON DRIED TARRAGON

Method

1. Trim ends from each leaf of artichoke with scissors.
2. Combine water, peppercorns, fennel seeds, and 1 tablespoon lemon juice in saucepan.
3. Bring to a boil; add artichoke. Reduce heat, cover tightly, and simmer over low heat until heart is easily pierced with tip of knife, about 45 minutes, turning once.
4. Whisk together remaining 1 teaspoon lemon juice, olive oil, and mustard; serve with artichoke for dipping.

Method-Microwave

1. Trim ends from each leaf of artichoke with scissors.
2. Combine water, peppercorns, fennel seeds, and 1 tablespoon lemon juice in large microwave-safe casserole dish or 2-quart glass measure.
3. Cover and cook on high power until boiling, about 3 minutes. Add artichoke; cook on high power 1 minute. Reduce power to medium and continue to cook 13–15 minutes or until heart is easily pierced with tip of knife, turning artichoke over halfway through cooking. Let stand covered 5 minutes.
4. Prepare sauce as in step 4 above.

Custard-Style Corn Pudding

Yield: 6 servings
Serving Size: ⅙ recipe
Exchanges:

		Nutrient Content per Serving		
		CAL	116	Na	139 (mg)
		PRO	9 (gm)	K	333 (mg)
Starch/Bread	0.5	Fat	2.1 (gm)	Fiber	2 (gm)
Milk, skim	1.0	CHO	17 (gm)	Chol	3 (mg)

Ingredients

½ CUP FINELY CHOPPED ONION
1 TABLESPOON MARGARINE
¾ CUP EGG SUBSTITUTE
1½ CUPS FROZEN WHOLE KERNEL CORN, THAWED
1 12-OUNCE CAN EVAPORATED SKIM MILK (1½ CUPS)

Method

1. Preheat over to 350°F.
2. Sauté onion in margarine until tender, about 5 minutes.
3. Combine egg substitute, corn, and milk; stir in onion mixture. Pour into 9-inch pie plate.
4. Place plate in large shallow pan of hot water. Bake 35–40 minutes or until a knife inserted near center comes out clean. Serve warm.

Artichoke and Tomato Sauté

Yield: 4 servings

Serving Size: ¼ recipe

Exchanges:

Vegetable   1.0

Fat   0.5

Nutrient Content per Serving

CAL	51	Na	112 (mg)
PRO	2 (gm)	K	259 (mg)
Fat	2.1 (gm)	Fiber	1.3 (gm)
CHO	7 (gm)	Chol	0 (mg)

Ingredients

   1 6-OUNCE JAR MARINATED ARTICHOKE HEARTS
   1 SMALL RED ONION, CUT INTO THIN WEDGES
   1 CLOVE GARLIC, MINCED
   1 LARGE TOMATO, SEEDED AND CHOPPED
  ¼ TEASPOON SHREDDED LEMON PEEL
    LEMON WEDGES
    FRESHLY GROUND BLACK PEPPER

Method

1. Spoon off 1 tablespoon oil from top of artichoke marinade into 10-inch skillet. Sauté onion and garlic in oil until softened, about 4 minutes.
2. Drain remaining marinade from artichokes; add artichokes to skillet with tomato and lemon peel. Sauté until heated through, about 2 minutes. Serve with lemon wedges and pepper.

Method-Microwave

1. Spoon off 1 tablespoon oil from top of artichoke marinade into shallow 1½-quart casserole dish. Toss onion and garlic with oil. Cover and cook on high power 3–4 minutes.
2. Drain remaining marinade from artichokes; add artichokes to dish with tomato and lemon peel. Cover and cook on high power 2–3 minutes or until heated through. Serve with lemon wedges and pepper.

Whipped Potatoes with Horseradish

Yield: 2-½ cups (5 servings)   Nutrient Content per Serving

Serving Size: ½ cup	CAL	130	Na	75 (mg)
Exchanges:	PRO	3 (gm)	K	351 (mg)
Starch/Bread	1.0	Fat	4.7 (gm)	Fiber	2 (gm)
Fat	1.0	CHO	20 (gm)	Chol	1 (mg)

Ingredients

- 2 LARGE BAKING POTATOES, PEELED AND CUT INTO 2-INCH CHUNKS (ABOUT 1¼ POUNDS)
- 2 TABLESPOONS MARGARINE
- ¼ CUP EVAPORATED SKIM MILK
- 1 TABLESPOON FRESHLY GRATED HORSERADISH OR DRAINED PREPARED HORSERADISH
- ¼ TEASPOON FRESHLY GROUND BLACK PEPPER

Method

1. Place potatoes in boiling water and cook until tender, about 15 minutes. Drain well.
2. With electric mixer (do not use food processor or potatoes will be pasty), whip hot potatoes with margarine and milk until light and fluffy.
3. Add horseradish and pepper; mix well. Serve immediately.

Poached Cucumbers

Yield: 2 cups (4 servings)	Nutrient Content per Serving			
Serving Size: ½ cup	CAL	41	*Na	42 (mg)
Exchanges:	PRO	1 (gm)	K	109 (mg)
Vegetable 1.0	Fat	3.1 (gm)	Fiber	0.8 (gm)
Fat 0.5	CHO	3 (gm)	Chol	0 (mg)

*Add 133 mg if optional salt is used.

Ingredients

1 LARGE CUCUMBER, UNPEELED, HALVED LENGTH-
WISE, AND SEEDED (14 OUNCES BEFORE SEEDING,
12 OUNCES AFTER SEEDING)
½ CUP REDUCED-SODIUM CHICKEN BROTH OR
HOMEMADE (PAGE 118)
1 TABLESPOON MARGARINE
¼ TEASPOON SALT (OPTIONAL)
FRESHLY GROUND BLACK PEPPER

Method

1. Slice cucumber ¼ inch thick. Combine cucumber and broth in medium saucepan. Cover and simmer over low heat until tender, about 4–5 minutes.
2. Drain and discard liquid. Toss with margarine until melted. Sprinkle with salt, if desired. Serve with pepper.

Method-Microwave

1. Slice cucumber ¼ inch thick. Combine cucumber and broth in shallow microwave-safe casserole. Cover with vented plastic wrap. Cook on high power 5–7 minutes or until tender.
2. Drain and discard liquid. Toss with margarine until melted. Sprinkle with salt, if desired. Serve with pepper.

Braised Endive

Yield: 2 servings	Nutrient Content per Serving			
Serving Size: 1 whole endive	CAL	29	Na	58 (mg)
Exchanges:	PRO	1 (gm)	K	121 (mg)
Vegetable 1.0	Fat	0.6 (gm)	Fiber	1.1 (gm)
	CHO	5 (gm)	Chol	0 (mg)

Ingredients

    2 WHOLE BELGIAN ENDIVE (8 OUNCES)
    ½ CUP REDUCED-SODIUM CHICKEN BROTH
    1 TEASPOON DIJON-STYLE MUSTARD
    1 TEASPOON HONEY
      FRESHLY GROUND BLACK PEPPER

Method

1. Cut endive lengthwise in half.
2. Combine broth, mustard, and honey in saucepan large enough to hold endive in one layer. Bring to a boil. Add endive to broth cut side down; reduce heat. Cover and simmer until tender, about 5 minutes, basting once with liquid in saucepan.
3. Transfer endive and broth to shallow dish. Serve with pepper.

Method-Microwave

1. Cut endive lengthwise in half.
2. Whisk together broth, mustard, and honey in shallow microwave-safe dish large enough to hold endive in one layer. Add endive to broth cut side down; cover and cook on high power, 3 minutes. Baste endive with juices in dish. Cover and continue to cook until tender, 3–4 minutes. Serve with pepper.

Stir-Fry Bok Choy with Mirin

		Nutrient Content per Serving		
Yield: 2 cups (4 servings)				
Serving Size: ½ cup		CAL	39	Na 334 (mg)
Exchanges:		PRO	2 (gm)	K 383 (mg)
Vegetable	1.0	Fat	2.4 (gm)	Fiber 1.6 (gm)
Fat	0.5	CHO	3 (gm)	Chol 0 (mg)

Ingredients

> 1 SMALL HEAD BOK CHOY (1 POUND)
> 1 TEASPOON ORIENTAL SESAME OIL*
> 1 TEASPOON PEANUT OR VEGETABLE OIL*
> 2 TABLESPOONS REDUCED-SODIUM SOY SAUCE
> 2 TABLESPOONS MIRIN (SWEET RICE WINE)

Method

1. Slice large green leaves of bok choy into thin strips; set aside. Slice white stalks of bok choy ½ inch thick.
2. Heat both oils in large skillet or wok over medium-high heat. Stir-fry stalks until crisp-tender, 2–3 minutes. Add green leaves; stir-fry 1 minute more.
3. Add soy sauce and mirin; stir-fry about 1 minute. Serve immediately in shallow bowls with juices.

Method-Microwave

1. Prepare bok choy as in step 1 above.
2. Toss stalks with both oils in 2-quart microwave-safe dish. Cover and cook on high power 3 minutes. Stir in green leaves; cover and cook 1 minute more.
3. Stir in soy sauce and mirin, cook uncovered 2 minutes. Serve immediately.

*Two teaspoons Mild Oriental Flavored Oil (page 143) may be substituted for sesame and peanut oils, if desired.

Provençal Stuffed Eggplants

Yield: 4 servings
Serving Size: ½ stuffed
  eggplant
Exchanges:
Vegetable   3.0
Fat   0.5

Nutrient Content per Serving

CAL	94	*Na	19 (mg)
PRO	2 (gm)	K	524 (mg)
Fat	3.7 (gm)	Fiber	3.1 (gm)
CHO	15 (gm)	Chol	0 (mg)

*Add 133 mg if optional salt is used.

Ingredients

> 2 SMALL EGGPLANTS, 5–6 INCHES LONG (ABOUT 1½ POUNDS)
> NONSTICK VEGETABLE SPRAY
> 1 MEDIUM ONION, CHOPPED (6 OUNCES)
> 2 CLOVES GARLIC, MINCED
> 1 TABLESPOON OLIVE OIL
> 1 14½-OUNCE CAN NO-SALT-ADDED TOMATOES, DRAINED AND COARSELY CHOPPED
> ¼ CUP BASIL LEAVES, THINLY SLICED
> 1 TABLESPOON BALSAMIC OR RED WINE VINEGAR
> ¼ TEASPOON FRESHLY GROUND BLACK PEPPER
> ¼ TEASPOON SALT (OPTIONAL)

Method

1. Heat oven to 350°F.
2. Cut eggplants in half lengthwise. Spray cookie sheet with vegetable spray. Place eggplants cut side down on cookie sheet. Bake until tender when pierced with tip of knive, about 10–15 minutes.
3. Remove pulp from eggplant, leaving a ¼-inch shell. Coarsely chop eggplant.
4. Sauté onion and garlic in oil in skillet over medium heat under tender, about 5 minutes. Add eggplant; continue to sauté 3–4 minutes. Add tomatoes; cook 2 minutes. Stir in basil, vinegar, pepper and salt, if desired.
5. Spoon into eggplant shells; serve warm or at room temperature.

Method-Microwave

1. Cut eggplant in half lengthwise. Spray a shallow microwave-safe baking dish large enough to hold eggplant halves with cooking spray. Place eggplant cut side down in dish. Cover with waxed paper. Cook on high power 5–7 minutes or until tender when pierced with tip of knife.
2. Remove pulp from eggplant, leaving a ¼-inch shell. Coarsely chop eggplant.
3. Toss onion and garlic with oil in same baking dish. Cover with waxed paper. Cook on high power 3 minutes. Add eggplant; continue to cook 1–2 minutes. Add tomatoes; cover and cook 2 minutes. Stir in basil, vinegar, pepper and salt, if desired.

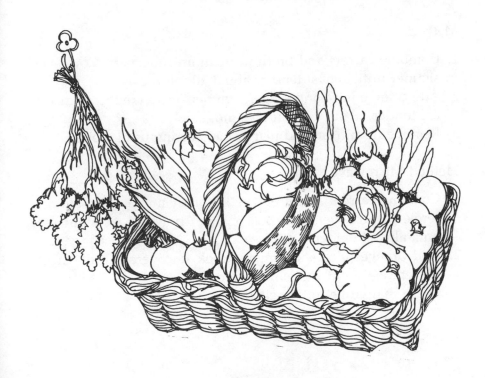

Gingered Orange Carrots

Yield: 2 cups (4 servings)
Serving Size: ½ cup
Exchanges:
Vegetable 1.0
Fat 0.5

Nutrient Content per Serving			
CAL	54	Na	67 (mg)
PRO	1 (gm)	K	164 (mg)
Fat	2.1 (gm)	Fiber	2 (gm)
CHO	8 (gm)	Chol	0 (mg)

Ingredients

    3 CUPS SLICED CARROTS (12 OUNCES)
    ¼ CUP REDUCED-SODIUM CHICKEN BROTH
    ¼ CUP ORANGE JUICE
    1 TEASPOON SHREDDED FRESH GINGER OR ¼ TEA-
    SPOON GROUND GINGER
    2 TEASPOONS MARGARINE

Method

1. Combine carrots and broth in medium saucepan. Cover and simmer until almost tender, about 10 minutes.
2. Add orange juice and ginger; simmer uncovered until carrots are tender, about 2–3 minutes more.
3. Remove from heat; add margarine, stirring until melted.

Method-Microwave

1. Combine carrots and broth in 1½-quart microwave-safe casserole dish. Cover and cook on high power 6–8 minutes or until almost tender.
2. Add orange juice and ginger. Cook uncovered until carrots are tender, about 2–3 minutes more.
3. Stir in margarine until melted.

Green Beans in Tarragon Cream

Yield: 4 servings
Serving Size: ¼ recipe
Exchanges:
Vegetable   1.0

Nutrient Content per Serving

CAL	25	Na	58 (mg)
PRO	2 (gm)	K	169 (mg)
Fat	0.3 (gm)	Fiber	1.6 (gm)
CHO	5 (gm)	Chol	0 (mg)

Ingredients

2 CUPS GREEN BEANS CUT IN 1-INCH PIECES
2 TABLESPOONS EVAPORATED SKIM MILK
1 TABLESPOON DIJON MUSTARD WITH TARRAGON
OR 1 TABLESPOON DIJON MUSTARD PLUS ½ TEA-
SPOON DRIED TARRAGON LEAVES

Method

1. Simmer green beans in small amount of water in covered saucepan until crisp-tender, about 6 minutes.
2. Transfer to colander to drain. Add milk and mustard to saucepan; cook and stir just until thickened, about 1 minute.
3. Return drained beans to saucepan; toss with sauce and serve immediately.

Method-Microwave

1. Place green beans in shallow microwave-safe casserole dish. Cover with vented plastic wrap. Cook on high power until crisp-tender, 2½–3 minutes.
2. Transfer to colander to drain. Add milk and mustard to dish, whisking to combine. Cook uncovered on high power 1–2 minutes or until heated through.
3. Return drained beans to dish; toss with sauce and serve immediately.

Pesto-Flavored Squash Sauté

Yield: 4 servings
Serving Size: ¼ recipe
Exchanges:
Vegetable 1.0
Fat 1.0

Nutrient Content per Serving

CAL	68	Na	27 (mg)
PRO	2 (gm)	K	175 (mg)
Fat	5.2 (gm)	Fiber	1.6 (gm)
CHO	5 (gm)	Chol	1 (mg)

Ingredients

> 1 TABLESPOON OLIVE OIL
> 1 MEDIUM ONION, CHOPPED
> 2 CLOVES GARLIC, MINCED
> 1 MEDIUM ZUCCHINI SQUASH, SLICED THIN
> 1 MEDIUM YELLOW SQUASH, SLICED THIN
> ¼ CUP BASIL LEAVES, MINCED
> 1 TABLESPOON PINE NUTS, TOASTED
> 1 TABLESPOON FRESHLY GRATED PARMESAN CHEESE
> FRESHLY GROUND BLACK PEPPER

Method

1. Heat oil in 10-inch skillet over medium heat. Sauté onion and garlic until tender, about 4 minutes. Add zucchini and yellow squash; toss. Cover and cook on high power 2–3 minutes or until crisp-tender.
2. Stir in basil; heat through. Sprinkle with pine nuts and cheese; serve with pepper.

Method-Microwave

1. Toss onion and garlic with oil in 2-quart microwave-safe casserole dish. Cook uncovered on high power 3 minutes. Add zucchini and yellow squash; toss. Cover and cook on high power 2–3 minutes or until crisp-tender.
2. Stir in basil; sprinkle with pine nuts and cheese. Serve with pepper.

Zucchini with Pepper and Cheese

		Nutrient Content per Serving		
Yield: 4 servings				
Serving Size: ¼ recipe		CAL 79	Na	115 (mg)
Exchanges:		PRO 4 (gm)	K	241 (mg)
Vegetable	1.0	Fat 5.8 (gm)	Fiber	2.7 (gm)
Fat	1.0	CHO 4 (gm)	Chol	10 (mg)

Ingredients

    1 TABLESPOON MARGARINE
    1 POUND ZUCCHINI SQUASH, SLICED ¼ INCH THICK
      (ABOUT 3½ CUPS)
 ¼–½ TEASPOON FRESHLY GROUND BLACK PEPPER, AS
      DESIRED
    ½ CUP (2 OUNCES) SHREDDED REDUCED-FAT MONTE-
      REY JACK CHEESE

Method

1. Heat margarine in large nonstick skillet. Sauté zucchini over medium-high heat until crisp-tender, about 4 minutes.
2. Sprinkle with pepper; toss well. Sprinkle evenly with cheese; remove from heat. Let stand covered until cheese melts, about 2 minutes.

Method-Microwave

1. Place margarine in shallow 1½-quart microwave-safe casserole dish. Cook on high power until melted, about 45 seconds. Toss zucchini in margarine. Cover with waxed paper; cook on high power until crisp-tender, about 4–5 minutes, rotating dish once.
2. Sprinkle with pepper; toss well. Sprinkle evenly with cheese; cook on high power until cheese melts, 30–60 seconds.

Grilled Cajun Corn on the Cob

Yield: 4 servings
Serving Size: ¼ recipe
Exchanges:
Starch/Bread   2.0
Fat   1.0

Nutrient Content per Serving

CAL	184	*Na	87 (mg)
PRO	4 (gm)	K	310 (mg)
Fat	7.3 (gm)	Fiber	5.8 (gm)
CHO	31 (gm)	Chol	0 (mg)

*Add 133 mg if optional salt is used.

Ingredients

   4 SWEET CORNCOBS WITH HUSK INTACT (12 OUNCES EACH)
   2 TABLESPOONS MARGARINE, SOFTENED
   ½ TEASPOON GARLIC POWDER
   ½ TEASPOON THYME
   ¼ TEASPOON FRESHLY GROUND BLACK PEPPER
   ¼ TEASPOON SALT (OPTIONAL)
   ⅛ TEASPOON CAYENNE (GROUND RED) PEPPER

Method

1. Peel back husks, but do not remove them. Remove and discard corn silk. Reclose husk around corncob; secure with twister seals or small pieces of wire. Soak in cold water to cover at least 20 minutes.
2. Grill drained corncobs on a covered grill over medium coals until steamed throughout, about 15–20 minutes, turning occasionally. While corn is grilling, combine remaining ingredients in small bowl. Husk hot corn and serve immediately with cajun mixture for spreading.

Note: If grill is not available, shuck corn and simmer in water to cover just until tender, about 6 minutes depending on maturity of corn. Drain and serve immediately with cajun mixture for spreading.

Stewed Sweet Peppers in Vinegar

Yield: 4 servings

Serving Size: ¼ recipe

Exchanges:

Vegetable   1.0

Fruit   0.5

Nutrient Content per Serving

CAL	61	Na	6 (mg)
PRO	1 (gm)	K	193 (mg)
Fat	0.3 (gm)	Fiber	3.4 (gm)
CHO	16 (gm)	Chol	0 (mg)

Ingredients

    1½ CUPS WATER
    ¼ CUP RASPBERRY VINEGAR (PAGE 147) OR BALSAMIC
        VINEGAR
    2 TABLESPOONS HONEY
    1 MEDIUM ONION, THINLY SLICED
    2 CLOVES GARLIC, SLICED
    6 WHOLE PEPPERCORNS
    1 BAY LEAF
    1 POUND RED OR YELLOW BELL PEPPERS, SEEDED
        AND CUT INTO WIDE STRIPS

Method

1. Combine water, vinegar, honey, onion, garlic, peppercorns, and bay leaf in medium saucepan. Bring to a boil.
2. Add peppers; simmer uncovered 15 minutes or until peppers are soft. Cool and refrigerate in liquid up to 1 week before serving. Serve chilled or at room temperature.

Method-Microwave

1. Combine water, vinegar, honey, onion, garlic, peppercorns, and bay leaf in shallow 1½-quart microwave-safe casserole dish. Cover and cook on high power until boiling, about 5 minutes.
2. Add peppers; cover and cook on medium power 16–18 minutes. Store and serve as in step 2 above.

Fresh Fennel Medley

Yield: 4 servings
Serving Size: ¼ recipe
Exchanges:
Vegetable   1.0
Fat   1.0

Nutrient Content per Serving

CAL	63	*Na	37 (mg)
PRO	1 (gm)	K	384 (mg)
Fat	3.7 (gm)	Fiber	2.0 (gm)
CHO	8 (gm)	Chol	0 (mg)

*Add 133 mg salt if desired.

Ingredients

1 MEDIUM BLUE FENNEL (10 OUNCES)
1 MEDIUM ONION, CUT INTO THIN WEDGES (USE SWEET ONION IF IN SEASON)
1 TABLESPOON OLIVE OIL
2 MEDIUM PLUM OR SMALL RIPE TOMATOES, CHOPPED
¼ TEASPOON SALT (OPTIONAL)
FRESHLY GROUND BLACK PEPPER

Method

1. Trim long stalks from fennel down to the bulb. Chop and reserve 2 tablespoons feathery green tops to fennel. Slice bulb; cut slices into strips.
2. Sauté fennel strips and onions in oil in small skillet until fennel is crisp-tender, 8–10 minutes. Stir in tomatoes and salt, if desired. Sprinkle with fennel tops and serve with pepper.

Method-Microwave

1. Prepare fennel as directed in step 1 above.
2. Toss fennel strips and onion with oil in 11-by-7-inch microwave-safe baking dish. Cover with vented plastic wrap and cook on high power 5–6 minutes or until fennel is crisp-tender, stirring once. Stir in tomato and salt, if desired. Cook uncovered on high power 1 minute. Sprinkle with fennel tops and serve with pepper.

Wild Mushrooms in Cognac

Yield: 2 cups (4 servings)   Nutrient Content per Serving

Serving Size: ½ cup

Exchanges:

		Nutrient Content per Serving			
CAL	61	Na	338 (mg)
PRO	2 (gm)	K	312 (mg)
Vegetable	2.0	Fat	3.1 (gm)	Fiber	2.6 (gm)
Fat	0.5	CHO	8 (gm)	Chol	0 (mg)

Ingredients

    1 OUNCE DRIED PORCINI, DRIED OR FRESH SHIITAKE,
       OR FRESH CHANTERELLE MUSHROOMS
    1 CLOVE GARLIC, MINCED
    1 TABLESPOON MARGARINE
    8 OUNCES BUTTON MUSHROOMS, SLICED
    ½ TEASPOON THYME
    2 TABLESPOONS BEEF BROTH OR STRAINED WATER
       FROM SOAKING MUSHROOMS
    1 TABLESPOON COGNAC OR BRANDY
       FRESHLY GROUND BLACK PEPPER

Method

1. Soak dried mushrooms in boiling water to cover 30 minutes. Drain and slice. (If using skiitake mushrooms, discard tough stems.)
2. Sauté garlic in margarine in nonstick skillet over medium heat 1 minute. Add both kinds of mushrooms. Sprinkle with thyme. Sauté until mushrooms give up liquid and most of liquid is absorbed, about 5 minutes. Add broth and cognac; continue cooking 2 minutes. Serve with pepper.

Note: This is a simple but elegant side dish that is a perfect accompaniment to beef or veal. Large supermarket produce sections stock dried mushrooms, or look in the Oriental market for dried Chinese black mushrooms (shiitake).

Oriental Grilled Mushrooms and Onions

Yield: 4 servings
Serving Size: ¼ recipe
Exchanges
Vegetable 1.0
Fat 2.0

Nutrient Content per Serving

CAL	118	Na	3 (mg)
PRO	1 (gm)	K	195 (mg)
Fat	10.6 (gm)	Fiber	1.9 (gm)
CHO	6 (gm)	Chol	0 (mg)

Ingredients

> 2 TABLESPOONS PEANUT OIL
> 1 TABLESPOON ORIENTAL SESAME OIL
> 2 CLOVES GARLIC, MINCED
> 1 TABLESPOON FINELY SHREDDED FRESH GINGERROOT
> 4 OUNCES BUTTON MUSHROOMS, STEMS TRIMMED
> 4 OUNCES FRESH SHIITAKE MUSHROOMS, STEMS REMOVED
> 4 GREEN ONIONS, CUT INTO 1-INCH LENGTHS

Method

1. Combine oils, garlic, and ginger in medium bowl.
2. Add remaining ingredients; toss to coat. Let stand at room temperature 30 minutes.
3. Thread mushrooms alternately with onions onto skewers. Grill or broil 6–8 inches from heat source, turning often and brushing with any remaining oil mixture until tender, 5–7 minutes.

Baked Acorn Squash

Yield: 4 servings
Serving Size: ½ squash
Exchanges:
Starch/Bread   1.0
Fat   1.0

Nutrient Content per Serving

CAL	124	Na	72 (mg)
PRO	1 (gm)	K	395 (mg)
Fat	5.8 (gm)	Fiber	4.1 (gm)
CHO	19 (gm)	Chol	0 (mg)

Ingredients

    2 SMALL ACORN SQUASH, 1 POUND EACH
    2 TABLESPOONS MARGARINE, MELTED
    2 TABLESPOONS DARK BROWN SUGAR
    ¼ TEASPOON CINNAMON
    ⅛–¼ TEASPOON GROUND CLOVES, AS DESIRED

Method

1. Heat oven to 375°F.
2. Cut squash in half crosswise. Remove seeds and spongy membrane. Place cut side down in shallow roasting pan or jelly-roll pan. Bake until fork-tender, about 50–60 minutes.
3. Turn squash cut side up. Combine margarine, sugar, cinnamon, and cloves; brush over cut surface of squash. Return to oven; bake 5 minutes.

Method-Microwave

1. Pierce squash in several places with tip of sharp knive. Place on paper towel and cook on high power 12–15 minutes or unitl just fork-tender, turning squash over after 7 minutes. Let stand 10 minutes.
2. Cut squash in half crosswise. Discard seeds. Place in shallow microwave-safe dish large enough to hold upright in one layer. Combine margarine, sugar, cinnamon, and cloves; brush over cut surface of squash. Cook on high power 2 minutes.

Desserts

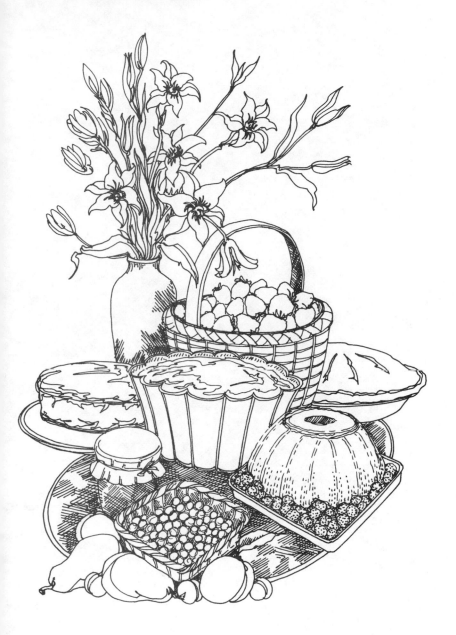

Light Rice Pudding

Yield: 2 cups (4 servings)
Serving Size: ½ cup
Exchanges:
Starch/Bread   1.5

Nutrient Content per Serving

CAL	116	Na	96 (mg)
PRO	3 (gm)	K	116 (mg)
Fat	0.2 (gm)	Fiber	0 (gm)
CHO	25 (gm)	Chol	1 (mg)

Ingredients

    1½ CUPS WATER
    ⅓ CUP ARBORIO OR SHORT-GRAIN RICE
    ⅛ TEASPOON SALT
    1 CUP SKIM MILK
    3 TABLESPOONS SUGAR
    2 TEASPOONS CORNSTARCH
    1 TEASPOON VANILLA
       GROUND NUTMEG OR CINNAMON

Method

1. Combine water, rice, and salt in medium saucepan. Bring to a
   boil. Reduce to a simmer. Cover and cook until rice is very
   tender, about 25 minutes.
2. Add milk. Combine sugar and cornstarch; slowly stir into rice
   mixture. Bring to a boil.
3. Boil gently until thickened, stirring constantly, about 2 minutes.
4. Remove from heat, stir in vanilla, and let cool to room temperature, stirring occasionally. Sprinkle with nutmeg or cinnamon as desired. Serve at room temperature or chilled.

Note: This dessert should be for occasional use only due to its
sugar content.

Ricotta-Filled Dessert Blintzes

Yield: 12 filled crêpes (6 servings)

Serving Size: 2 crêpes

Exchanges:

Starch/Bread	2.5
Meat, medium-fat	1.0

Nutrient Content per Serving

CAL	285	Na	176 (mg)
PRO	15 (gm)	K	218 (mg)
Fat	9.6 (gm)	Fiber	1 (gm)
CHO	35 (gm)	Chol	30 (mg)

Ingredients

Crêpes:

¾ CUP ALL-PURPOSE FLOUR
¾ CUP SKIM MILK
½ CUP EGG SUBSTITUTE OR 2 EGG WHITES
1 TABLESPOON MARGARINE, MELTED
    NONSTICK VEGETABLE SPRAY

Filling:

1 15-OUNCE CONTAINER LOW-FAT RICOTTA CHEESE
2 TABLESPOONS POWDERED SUGAR
1½ TEASPOONS PURE VANILLA
⅓ CUP STRAWBERRY OR RASPBERRY JAM OR CONSERVE

Method

1. Combine flour, milk, egg substitute, and margarine in food processor or blender. Process until smooth. Let stand at room temperature 1 hour or refrigerate up to 8 hours. Process 1 second before using.
2. Heat 5–6-inch crêpe pan over medium heat. Spray with nonstick vegetable spray.
3. Pour about 3 tablespoons batter (use ¼ cup dry measuring cup about ¾ full) into hot pan, tilting to spread batter evenly. Cook until bottom is lightly browned; turn and cook 30 seconds more.
4. Remove each crêpe to sheet of waxed paper and repeat process until all batter is used (12 crêpes).*

5. For filling, combine cheese, sugar, and vanilla in food processor or blender. Process until smooth.
6. Spoon 2 heaping tablespoons filling down center of each crêpe. Roll up; place seam side down in 11-by-7-inch glass baking dish that has been sprayed with vegetable spray.
7. Cover with foil.** Bake in 350°F oven 15–18 minutes or until heated through. Serve warm with jam.

Note: For quick, individual servings, sauté filled crêpes in nonstick skillet sprayed with vegetable spray.

    *Crêpes may be wrapped securely and frozen for up to 3 months or refrigerated for 2 days.
    **Filled crêpes may be refrigerated up to 24 hours before baking. Increase baking time to 20 minutes.

Quick Yogurt Dessert

Yield: 1 serving

Exchanges:

		Nutrient Content per Serving			
		CAL	142	Na	88 (mg)
Fruit	1.0	PRO	7 (gm)	K	316 (mg)
Milk, skim	1.0	Fat	2.0 (gm)	Fiber	1 (gm)
		CHO	24 (gm)	Chol	8 (mg)

Ingredients

    ½ CUP PLAIN LOW-FAT YOGURT
    2 TEASPOONS FRUIT PRESERVES OR CONSERVE
    2 TABLESPOONS COOKED AND CHILLED BROWN RICE

Method

1. Whisk together yogurt and preserves. Stir in rice.

Baked Papaya with Cinnamon

Yield: 2 servings
Serving Size: ½ payaya
Exchanges:
Fruit   1.0
Fat   0.5

Nutrient Content per Serving

	with brown sugar	with brown sugar substitute
CAL	93	78
PRO	1 (gm)	1 (gm)
Fat	2.1 (gm)	2.1 (gm)
CHO	19 (gm)	15 (gm)
Na	28 (mg)	26 (mg)
K	411 (mg)	396 (mg)
Fiber	2 (gm)	2 (gm)
Chol	0 (mg)	0 (mg)

Ingredients

    1 RIPE PAPAYA (1 POUND)
    2 TEASPOONS BROWN SUGAR OR BROWN SUGAR
      SUBSTITUTE
    1 TEASPOON SUNFLOWER MARGARINE, MELTED
    ⅛ TEASPOON GROUND CINNAMON

Method

1. Heat oven to 350°F.
2. Cut papaya in half lengthwise; scoop out and discard seeds. Place cut side up in shallow baking dish.
3. Combine sugar, margarine, and cinnamon; brush over cut sides of papaya.
4. Bake 15–20 minutes or until heated through. Serve warm or at room temperature.

Method-Microwave

1. Prepare papaya as in steps 1–3 above.
2. Cook uncovered on high power 3–4 minutes or until heated through.
3. Let stand 5 minutes. Serve warm or at room temperature.

Note: Ripe papayas are a rich yellow color with just a hint of green. If the papaya is purchased green, store in a paper bag at room temperature several days or until yellow.

Tropical Fruit Cup

Yield: 2 cups (4 servings)	Nutrient Content per Serving			
Serving Size: ½ cup	CAL	61	Na	2 (mg)
Exchanges:	PRO	1 (gm)	K	184 (mg)
Fruit 1.0	Fat	0.3 (gm)	Fiber	2 (gm)
	CHO	16 (gm)	Chol	0 (mg)

Ingredients

    1 CUP RIPE PAPAYA CHUNKS (4 OUNCES)
    1 CUP FRESH PINEAPPLE CUBES (4 OUNCES)
    ½ CUP RIPE MANGO CHUNKS (4 OUNCES)
    1 TABLESPOON ORANGE-FLAVORED LIQUEUR
    1 TEASPOON FRESH LIME JUICE
        LIME WEDGES

Method

1. Combine fruit in serving bowl.
2. Pour liqueur and lime juice over fruit; toss lightly to coat. Serve immediately or cover and chill up to 6 hours. Serve with lime wedges.

Note: Serve this cool and refreshing dessert after a spicy meal.

Sautéed Spiced Apples

Yield: 1½ cups (2 servings)   Nutrient Content per Serving
Serving Size: ¾ cup

Exchanges:	CAL	159	Na	48 (mg)
	PRO	0 (gm)	K	226 (mg)
Fruit 2.0	Fat	4.4 (gm)	Fiber	3 (gm)
Fat 1.0	CHO	33 (gm)	Chol	0 (mg)

Ingredients

- 1 LARGE (OR 2 SMALL) GRANNY SMITH OR OTHER TART APPLE (ABOUT 12 OUNCES)
- 2 TABLESPOONS UNSWEETENED APPLE JUICE
- 1 TABLESPOON BROWN SUGAR OR BROWN SUGAR SUBSTITUTE*
- 2 TEASPOONS MARGARINE
- ¼ TEASPOON GROUND CINNAMON
- ⅛ TEASPOON NUTMEG, PREFERABLY FRESHLY GRATED

Method

1. Core apple but do not peel. Slice thinly.
2. Heat apple juice, sugar, and margarine in large nonstick skillet over medium heat.
3. Add apples; sprinkle with cinnamon and nutmeg. Cook and stir until most of liquid is evaporated and apples are tender, about 5 minutes. Serve warm, at room temperature, or chilled.

Method-Microwave

1. Core apple but do not peel. Slice thinly.
2. Toss apple, apple juice, sugar, margarine, cinnamon, and nutmeg in shallow microwave-safe dish.
3. Cook on high power 4–6 minutes or until apples are tender, stirring twice. Serve warm, at room temperature, or chilled.

*Brown sugar substitute will reduce calories and carbohydrate slightly, but will not change exchange values.

Quick Raspberry Ice

Yield: 1 cup (2 servings)	Nutrient Content per Serving			
Serving Size: ½ cup	CAL	122	Na	2 (mg)
Exchanges:	PRO	2 (gm)	K	288 (mg)
Fruit 2.0	Fat	0.4 (gm)	Fiber	2 (gm)
	CHO	27 (gm)	Chol	0 (mg)

Ingredients

    2 CUPS FROZEN UNSWEETENED RASPBERRIES
    1 TABLESPOON ORANGE LIQUEUR
      MINT SPRIGS (OPTIONAL)

Method

1. Place raspberries and liqueur in food processor fitted with steel blade.
2. Process until thick and smooth, scraping down sides once. Serve immediately garnished with mint sprig, if desired.

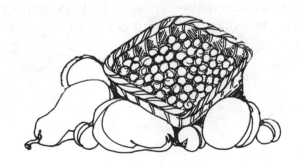

Port Poached Pears

Yield: 2 servings
Serving Size: ½ poached pear
Exchanges:
Fruit   1.0

Nutrient Content per Serving

CAL	63	Na	3 (mg)
PRO	0 (gm)	K	132 (mg)
Fat	0.3 (gm)	Fiber	3 (gm)
CHO	16 (gm)	Chol	0 (mg)

Ingredients

    1 LARGE FIRM BUT RIPE PEAR, PEELED AND CORED
    ½ CUP PORT WINE
      FRESHLY GROUND BLACK PEPPER (OPTIONAL)

Method

1. Preheat oven to 350°F.
2. Place pear halves cut side down in small glass pie plate or ovenproof casserole. Pour wine over pear.
3. Bake uncovered 20–30 minutes or until pear is tender when pierced with tip of knife, basting each 10 minutes. Cooking time will vary depending on ripeness of pear. Let stand in pie plate until cooled to room temperature, spooning port over pear several times.
4. Transfer to dessert dishes; spoon 1 tablespoon port over each pear half, discarding remaining port. Garnish with pepper, if desired.

Fresh Peach Cobbler

Yield: 8 servings
Serving Size: ⅛ recipe
Exchanges:

Starch/Bread	1.0
Fruit	1.0
Fat	1.0

Nutrient Content per Serving

CAL	181	Na	69 (mg)
PRO	2 (gm)	K	261 (mg)
Fat	6.3 (gm)	Fiber	2 (gm)
CHO	30 (gm)	Chol	0 (mg)

Ingredients

> 6 CUPS FRESH PEELED AND SLICED PEACHES (ABOUT
> 6 MEDIUM PEACHES OR 2 POUNDS)
> 2 TABLESPOONS ALMOND-FLAVORED LIQUEUR
> ½ TEASPOON CINNAMON
> DASH OF FRESHLY GRATED NUTMEG
> ¾ CUP QUICK-COOKING OATS, UNCOOKED
> ¼ CUP ALL-PURPOSE FLOUR
> ⅓ CUP LIGHT BROWN SUGAR*
> ¼ CUP MARGARINE, CHILLED, CUT INTO 4 PIECES

Method

1. Preheat oven to 375°F.
2. Combine peaches, liqueur, cinnamon, and nutmeg. Spoon into 8-inch square glass baking dish or 10-inch deep-dish pie plate.
3. Combine oats, flour, and sugar. Cut in margarine until crumbly; sprinkle over peaches. Bake 30 minutes or until peaches are tender and topping is golden brown. Serve warm or at room temperature.

*For occasional use due to sugar content.

Meringue Cookies

Yield: 3 dozen	Nutrient Content per Serving			
Serving Size: 2 cookies	CAL	32	Na	13 (mg)
Exchanges:	PRO	1 (gm)	K	11 (mg)
Fruit 0.5	Fat	1.1 (gm)	Fiber	0 (gm)
	CHO	5 (gm)	Chol	0 (mg)

Ingredients

    2 LARGE EGG WHITES
    ¾ CUP POWDERED SUGAR
    1 TEASPOON VANILLA
      DASH OF SALT
    1 OUNCE TOASTED CHOPPED PECANS OR
      UNBLANCHED ALMONDS (⅓ CUP)
      NONSTICK VEGETABLE COOKING SPRAY

Method

1. Preheat oven to 300°F.
2. Beat egg whites with electric mixer until frothy.
3. Slowly beat in sugar, mixing well after each addition; continue beating at medium-high speed until stiff peaks form.
4. Fold in vanilla and salt, then nuts.
5. Spray cookie sheet with vegetable cooking spray.
6. Drop by teaspoons onto cookie sheet. Shape with back of spoon into 1-inch circles. Bake until golden brown and crisp, about 18–20 minutes. Immediately transfer to wire rack to cool.

Note: These flourless cookies are perfect for wheat-free diets and at Passover time. Store between sheets of waxed paper loosely covered at room temperature. Do not attempt to make in damp weather.

Creamy Cheese and Berry Bars

Yield: 4 servings
Serving Size: 2 bars
Exchanges:
Starch/Bread   1.0
Meat, medium-fat   1.0

Nutrient Content per Serving

CAL	134	Na	46 (mg)
PRO	6 (gm)	K	210 (mg)
Fat	4.5 (gm)	Fiber	3 (gm)
CHO	18 (gm)	Chol	16 (mg)

Ingredients

- ½ CUP LOW-FAT RICOTTA CHEESE (4 OUNCES)
- 1 OUNCE NEUFCHÂTEL CHEESE, CUBED, SOFTENED
- 1 TABLESPOON HONEY
- 1 TABLESPOON CHOPPED FRESH MINT LEAVES (OPTIONAL)
- 8 PIECES CRISPBREAD OR OTHER SNACKBREAD WAFERS (ABOUT 4-BY-2 INCHES, ½ OUNCE EACH)
- 2 CUPS SLICED STRAWBERRIES (8 OUNCES) MINT SPRIGS (OPTIONAL)

Method

1. Whip cheeses with electric mixer until smooth. Beat in honey. Fold in mint leaves, if desired.
2. Spread crackers with cheese mixture; arrange strawberries over cheese. Garnish with mint sprig, if desired. Serve immediately.

Rhubarb Compote

Yield: 1¾ cups (4 servings)	Nutrient Content per Serving			
Serving Size: ¼ recipe	CAL	80	Na	3 (mg)
Exchanges:	PRO	1 (gm)	K	184 (mg)
Fruit 1.0	Fat	0.2 (gm)	Fiber	1.5 (gm)
	CHO	17 (gm)	Chol	0 (mg)

Ingredients

  1 CUP SLICED FRESH OR THAWED FROZEN RHUBARB
    (4 OUNCES)
  ½ CUP UNSWEETENED WHITE GRAPE JUICE
  1 TABLESPOON HONEY
  ½ CUP SLICED STRAWBERRIES (4 OUNCES)
  2 TABLESPOONS CASSIS LIQUEUR

Method

1. Simmer rhubarb in grape juice and honey uncovered until tender, about 10 minutes for fresh rhubarb, 5 minutes for frozen. Cool to room temperature.
2. Stir in strawberries; divide among dessert bowls. Serve at room temperature or chilled. Drizzle with liqueur just before serving.

Method-Microwave

1. Combine rhubarb, grape juice, and honey in 1-quart microwave-safe dish. Cook uncovered on high power until tender, about 6–8 minutes for fresh rhubarb, 4–6 minutes for forzen. Cool to room temperature.
2. Serve as above in step 2.

Fresh Fruit Clafouti

Yield: 4 servings
Serving Size: ¼ recipe
Exchanges:
Fruit   2.0

Nutrient Content per Serving

CAL	119	Na	133 (mg)
PRO	6 (gm)	K	318 (mg)
Fat	0.5 (gm)	Fiber	1.2 (gm)
CHO	24 (gm)	*Chol	2 (mg)

*Add 69 mg if whole egg is used.

Ingredients

    NONSTICK VEGETABLE SPRAY
 1½ CUPS SLICED RIPE NECTARINES, PLUMS, OR PEACHES
     (ABOUT 10 OUNCES)
 ⅔ CUP EVAPORATED SKIM MILK
 ¼ CUP EGG SUBSTITUTE OR 1 EGG, BEATEN
 2 TABLESPOONS FLOUR
 2 TABLESPOONS GRANULATED SUGAR
 ½ TEASPOON VANILLA
 ⅛ TEASPOON NUTMEG, PREFERABLY FRESHLY GRATED
 ⅛ TEASPOON SALT
 1 TABLESPOON SIFTED POWDERED SUGAR

Method

1. Heat oven to 375°F. Spray 8-inch glass pie plate with cooking spray. Layer fruit in pie plate.
2. Combine milk, egg, flour, sugar, vanilla, nutmeg, and salt in food processor fitted with steel blade. Process until smooth; pour over fruit.
3. Bake 35–40 minutes or until puffed and golden brown. Sprinkle with powdered sugar; serve warm or at room temperature.

Note: This dessert makes a nice addition to a brunch menu.

Lemony Poppy Seed Cake

Yield: 9 servings

Serving Size: 3-inch square piece of cake

Exchanges:

Starch/Bread 2.0

Fat 1.0

Nutrient Content per Serving

CAL	184	Na	204 (mg)
PRO	4 (gm)	K	91 (mg)
Fat	7.4 (gm)	Fiber	0.9 (gm)
CHO	26 (gm)	Chol	0 (mg)

Ingredients

NONSTICK VEGETABLE COOKING SPRAY
1 CUP FLOUR
½ CUP GRANULATED SUGAR
⅓ CUP POPPY SEEDS
1½ TEASPOONS BAKING POWDER
½ TEASPOON BAKING SODA
⅛ TEASPOON SALT
¼ CUP MARGARINE, MELTED
¼ CUP EGG SUBSTITUTE OR 2 EGG WHITES
½ CUP SKIM MILK
3 TABLESPOONS FRESH LEMON JUICE
1 TEASPOON FINELY GRATED LEMON PEEL
½ TEASPOON VANILLA
2 TABLESPOONS SIFTED POWDERED SUGAR

Method

1. Preheat oven to 350°F. Spray 9-inch square baking pan with vegetable spray.
2. Combine flour, granulated sugar, poppy seeds, baking powder, and baking soda in large bowl.
3. Add margarine, egg substitute, milk, lemon juice, zest, and vanilla. Mix just until dry ingredients are moistened. Pour into prepared pan. Bake 30 minutes or until cake springs back when center is lightly pressed.
4. Cool. Sprinkle with powdered sugar. Cut into squares to serve.

Hawaiian Soufflé Meal Pudding

Yield: 8 cups (8 servings)		Nutrient Content per Serving		
Serving Size: 1 cup		CAL	202	Na	180 (mg)
Exchanges:		PRO	6 (gm)	K	292 (mg)
Starch/Bread	2.0	Fat	5.7 (gm)	Fiber	3.4 (gm)
Fat	1.0	CHO	32 (gm)	Chol	1 (mg)

Ingredients

NONSTICK VEGETABLE COOKING SPRAY
2 CUPS ORANGE JUICE
1 CUP WHITE CORNMEAL
¼ TEASPOON SALT
2 TABLESPOONS MARGARINE
1 CUP EVAPORATED SKIM MILK
1 TEASPOON VANILLA
4 EGG WHITES, BEATEN TO STIFF PEAKS
3 TABLESPOONS GRANULATED SUGAR
1 CUP FLAKED COCONUT (2 OUNCES)

Method

1. Heat oven to 400°F. Spray 1½-quart soufflé dish with cooking spray.
2. Combine orange juice, cornmeal, and salt in saucepan. Bring to a boil, whisking constantly. Reduce heat; add margarine. Cook and stir until thickened, about 5 minutes.
3. Remove from heat; slowly whisk in milk and vanilla.
4. Beat egg whites.
5. Stir in sugar and coconut. Mix well. Fold in egg whites.
6. Pour mixture in soufflé dish; bake 30 minutes. Reduce oven temperature to 325°F and continue baking 15 minutes or until puffed and dark golden brown. Cool 15 minutes. (Soufflé will fall.) Serve warm or chilled.

Note: This delicious dessert keeps well refrigerated and is a big hit with children as well as adults.

Oranges with Southern-Style Bourbon Syrup

Yield: 4 servings

Serving Size: ¼ recipe

Exchanges:

Fruit　　1.0

Nutrient Content per Serving

CAL	62	Na	0 (mg)
PRO	1 (gm)	K	148 (mg)
Fat	0.1 (gm)	Fiber	1.3 (gm)
CHO	16 (gm)	Chol	0 (mg)

Ingredients

　　2 LARGE NAVEL ORANGES (1 POUND)
　　½ CUP WATER
　　2 TABLESPOONS SUGAR
　　1 TABLESPOON BOURBON WHISKEY OR IRISH WHISKEY

Method

1. Cut wide, thin strips of peel (colored part only) from one orange using a vegetable peeler. Cut into long, thin strips.
2. Combine water and sugar in small saucepan. Cook uncovered until sugar dissolves. Add peel; simmer uncovered 3–4 minutes. Add bourbon; continue to simmer 1 minute. Cool.
3. Cut all peel and white pith from oranges. Slice thinly and place in shallow serving bowl. Pour syrup over oranges. Chill until cold.

Method-Microwave

1. Cut peel from orange as directed in step 1 above.
2. Combine hot tap water and sugar in 1-cup glass measure. Stir in peel. Cook uncovered on high power 1½ minutes. Reduce power to medium and cook 2–3 minutes. Add bourbon; continue cooking 1 minute. Cool.
3. Prepare oranges as in step 3 above.

Peaches with Fresh Banana Sauce

	Nutrient Content per Serving			
Yield: 4 servings				
Serving Size: 2 tablespoons	CAL	66	Na	1 (mg)
sauce plus ½ cup peaches	PRO	1 (gm)	K	296 (mg)
Exchanges:	Fat	0.2 (gm)	Fiber	1.9 (gm)
Fruit 1.0	CHO	17 (gm)	Chol	0 (mg)

Ingredients

   1 RIPE MEDIUM BANANA (6 OUNCES)
   2 TABLESPOONS ORANGE JUICE
   1 TEASPOON FINELY SHREDDED ORANGE PEEL
   2 CUPS SLICED UNPEELED PEACHES OR NECTARINES
      FRESHLY GRATED NUTMEG

Method

1. Peel and break banana into large chunks. Place in blender container with orange juice and peel.
2. Blend until smooth, scraping down sides once. Serve immediately over sliced peaches; sprinkle with nutmeg.

Variation: For spirited banana sauce, substitute 1 tablespoon orange-flavored liqueur for 1 tablespoon orange juice.

Spiced Apple Coffee Cake

Yield: 9 servings
Serving Size: 2-inch square piece of cake
Exchanges:
Starch/Bread 1.5
Fruit 1.0
Fat 1.0

Nutrient Content per Serving

CAL	228	Na	263 (mg)
PRO	4 (gm)	K	138 (mg)
Fat	5.6 (gm)	Fiber	1.6 (gm)
CHO	40 (gm)	Chol	1 (mg)

Ingredients

NONSTICK VEGETABLE COOKING SPRAY
½ CUP BROWN SUGAR
¼ CUP MARGARINE, SOFTENED
2 EGG WHITES
½ CUP LOW-FAT BUTTERMILK
2 CUPS ALL-PURPOSE FLOUR
2 TEASPOONS BAKING POWDER
½ TEASPOON BAKING SODA
2 TEASPOONS CINNAMON
¼ TEASPOON SALT
1 MEDIUM APPLE, UNPEELED AND FINELY CHOPPED
(1 CUP)

Method

1. Heat oven to 375°F. Spray 9-by-9-inch baking pan with vegetable spray.
2. Beat together sugar, margarine, and egg whites until smooth. Stir in buttermilk. Add combined dry ingredients, mixing just until dry ingredients are moistened. (Batter will be stiff.) Fold in apple; spread in prepared pan.
3. Bake 25–30 minutes or until toothpick inserted in center comes out clean. Serve warm or at room temperature.

Northwest Berry Puff

Yield: 6 servings
Serving Size: ⅙ recipe
Exchanges:
Starch/Bread   1.0
Fat   0.5

Nutrient Content per Serving
CAL   108   Na   89 (mg)
PRO   5 (gm)   K   146 (mg)
Fat   2.2 (gm)   Fiber   2.5 (gm)
CHO   17 (gm)   Chol   92 (mg)

Ingredients

    NONSTICK VEGETABLE COOKING SPRAY
    2 WHOLE EGGS
    1 EGG WHITE
    ½ CUP SKIM MILK
    ½ CUP ALL-PURPOSE FLOUR
    1 TABLESPOON GRANULATED SUGAR
    ⅛ TEASPOON SALT
    2 CUPS FRESH RASPBERRIES, BLACKBERRIES, BOYSEN-
      BERRIES, BLUEBERRIES, SLICES STRAWBERRIES, OR
      A COMBINATION
    1 TABLESPOON SIFTED POWDERED SUGAR
    1 LEMON, CUT INTO 6 WEDGES

Method

1. Heat oven to 450°F. Spray 10-inch ovenproof skillet or Pyrex
   pie plate with vegetable spray.
2. Beat eggs and egg white in medium bowl. Whisk in milk.
   Slowly whisk in flour, granulated sugar, and salt. Pour in
   prepared skillet. Bake 15 minutes. Reduce heat to 350°F and
   continue to bake 10 minutes or until puffed and brown.
3. Add fruit; sprinkle with powdered sugar. Cut into wedges;
   serve with lemon wedges.

Melon Balls in Amaretto with Mint

Yield: 4 servings
Serving Size: 1 cup
Exchanges:
Fruit   1.5

Nutrient Content per Serving

CAL	102	Na	17 (mg)
PRO	1 (gm)	K	482 (mg)
Fat	0.3 (gm)	Fiber	1.5 (gm)
CHO	21 (gm)	Chol	0 (mg)

Ingredients

- 2 CUPS HONEYDEW MELON BALLS OR CHUNKS (8 OUNCES)
- 2 CUPS CANTALOUPE OR CRENSHAW MELON BALLS OR CHUNKS (8 OUNCES)
- 3 TABLESPOONS AMARETTO (ALMOND-FLAVORED) LIQUEUR
- 2 TABLESPOONS CHOPPED FRESH MINT LEAVES MINT SPRIGS (OPTIONAL)

Method

1. Combine melon balls in medium bowl.
2. Toss with amaretto and mint; cover and refrigerate at least 1 hour or up to 6 hours. Toss before serving. Garnish with mint sprigs, if desired.

Poached Dried Fruit Compote

Yield: 2 cups (6 servings)
Serving Size: ⅓ cup
Exchanges:
Fruit   2.0

Nutrient Content per Serving

CAL	109	Na	14 (mg)
PRO	1 (gm)	K	343 (mg)
Fat	0.2 (gm)	Fiber	6.8 (gm)
CHO	29 (gm)	Chol	0 (mg)

Ingredients

    1 8-OUNCE PACKAGE MIXED DRIED FRUIT
    1 CUP WATER
    1 CUP SWEET WHITE WINE SUCH AS RIESLING OR
        RHINE
    1 CINNAMON STICK
    4 WHOLE CLOVES
    4 ALLSPICE OR JUNIPER BERRIES (OPTIONAL)

Method

1. Combine all ingredients in medium saucepan. Bring to a boil. Reduce heat, cover, and simmer until fruit is tender, about 15 minutes.
2. Refrigerate until chilled. Discard spices; serve in shallow bowls with liquid.

Method-Microwave

1. Combine all ingredients in 1½-quart microwave-safe dish. Cover tightly and cook on high power until simmering, about 6 minutes. Stir; reduce power to medium and cook until fruit is tender, 10–12 minutes.
2. Continue as directed in step 2 above.

Note: This recipe can be made with 8 ounces of one kind of dried fruit such as prunes or apricots. It will keep up to 5 days refrigerated.

Key Largo Bananas Flambé

Yield: 2 servings
Serving Size: ½ recipe
Exchanges:
Fruit   2.0
Fat   1.0

Nutrient Content per Serving

CAL	160	Na	70 (mg)
PRO	1 (gm)	K	388 (mg)
Fat	6.2 (gm)	Fiber	1.8 (gm)
CHO	28 (gm)	Chol	0 (mg)

Ingredients

    2 SMALL RIPE BUT FIRM BANANAS
    1 LIME WEDGE
    1 TABLESPOON MARGARINE
    1 TABLESPOON BROWN SUGAR
    2 TABLESPOONS RUM

Method

1. Peel bananas and slice in half lengthwise. Squeeze lime wedge over.
2. Melt margarine in nonstick skillet over medium heat. Sauté bananas 2 minutes per side. Sprinkle with brown sugar; cook 1 minute more per side.
3. Drizzle with rum; remove from stove and carefully ignite. Shake skillet until flames are extinguished. Serve immediately.

Berries with Gingered Peach Sauce

Yield: 2 servings
Serving Size: ½ recipe
Exchanges:
Fruit   2.0

Nutrient Content per Serving

CAL	113	Na	1 (mg)
PRO	1 (gm)	K	316 (mg)
Fat	0.6 (gm)	Fiber	8.2 (gm)
CHO	24 (gm)	Chol	0 (mg)

Ingredients

1 LARGE VERY RIPE PEACH, PEELED AND PITTED
1 TABLESPOON ALMOND-FLAVORED LIQUEUR
1 TEASPOON FINELY SHREDDED FRESH GINGER
1½ CUPS FRESH RASPBERRIES

Method

1. Cut peach into large chunks; place in blender container or food processor. Add liqueur and ginger; blend or process until smooth, scraping down sides as necessary.
2. Top berries with peach sauce; serve immediately.

Note: A tasty and very high fiber dessert.

Appendix: Exchange Lists for Meal Planning

Lists are based on principles of good nutrition that apply to everyone. Copyright © 1989 American Diabetes Association, The American Dietetic Association.

1   STARCH/BREAD LIST

Each item in this list contains approximately 15 grams of carbohydrate, 3 grams of protein, a trace of fat, and 80 calories. Whole grain products average about 2 grams of fiber per exchange. Some foods are higher in fiber. Those foods that contain 3 or more grams of fiber per exchange are footnoted.

You can choose your starch exchanges from any of the items on this list. If you want to eat a starch food that is not on this list, the general rule is that:

- ½ cup of cereal, grain, or pasta is one exchange
- 1 ounce of a bread product is one exchange

Your dietitian can help you be more exact.

CEREALS/GRAINS/PASTA

Bran cereals*, concentrated (such as Bran Buds®, All Bran®)	⅓ cup
Bran cereals*, flaked	½ cup
Bulgur (cooked)	½ cup
Cooked cereals	½ cup
Cornmeal (dry)	2½ Tbsp.
Grape-Nuts®	3 Tbsp.
Grits (cooked)	½ cup
Other ready-to-eat unsweetened cereals	¾ cup
Pasta (cooked)	½ cup
Puffed cereal	1½ cups
Rice, white or brown (cooked)	⅓ cup
Shredded wheat	½ cup
Wheat germ*	3 Tbsp.

*3 grams or more of fiber per exchange.

DRIED BEANS/PEAS/LENTILS

Beans* and peas* (cooked), such as kidney, white, split, black-eyed	⅓ cup
Lentils* (cooked)	⅓ cup
Baked beans*	¼ cup

*3 grams or more of fiber per exchange.

STARCHY VEGETABLES

Corn*	½ cup
Corn on cob*, 6 in. long	1
Lima beans*	½ cup
Peas, green* (canned or frozen)	½ cup

Plantain*	½ cup	
Potato, baked	1	small (3 oz)
Potato, mashed	½ cup	
Squash, winter* (acorn, butternut)	1 cup	
Yam, sweet potato, plain	⅓ cup	

*3 grams or more of fiber per exchange.

BREAD

Bagel	½ (1 oz.)
Bread sticks, crisp, 4 in. long × ½ in.	2 (⅔ oz.)
Croutons, low-fat	1 cup
English muffin	½
Frankfurter or hamburger bun	½ (1 oz.)
Pita, 6 in. across	½
Plain roll, small	1 (1 oz.)
Raisin, unfrosted	1 slice (1 oz.)
Rye, pumpernickel	1 slice (1 oz.)
Tortilla, 6 in. across	1
White (including French, Italian)	1 slice (1 oz.)
Whole wheat	1 slice (1 oz.)

CRACKERS/SNACKS

Animal crackers	8
Graham crackers, 2½ in. square	3
Matzoh	¾ oz.
Melba toast	5 slices
Oyster crackers	24
Popcorn (popped, no fat added	3 cups
Pretzels	¾ oz.

Ry-Krisp*, 2 in. × 3½ in.	4
Saltine-type crackers	6
Whole wheat crackers*, no fat added (crisp breads, such as Finn®, Kavli®, Wasa®)	2–4 slices (¾ oz.)

*3 grams or more of fiber per exchange.

STARCH FOODS PREPARED WITH FAT

(Count as 1 starch/bread exchange, plus 1 fat exchange.)

Biscuit, 2½ in. across	1
Chow mein noodles	½ cup
Corn bread, 2 in. cube	1 (2 oz.)
Cracker, round butter-type	6
French fried potatoes, 2 in. to 3½ in. long	10 (1½ oz.)
Muffin, plain, small	1
Pancake, 4 in. across	2
Stuffing, bread (prepared)	¼ cup
Taco shell, 6 in. across	2
Waffle, 4½ in. square	1
Whole wheat cracker*, fat added (such as Triscuits®)	4–6 (1 oz.)

*3 grams or more of fiber per exchange.

2 MEAT LIST

Each serving of meat and substitutes on this list contains about 7 grams of protein. The amount of fat and number of calories vary, depending on what kind of meat or substitute you choose. The list is divided into three parts based on the amount of fat and calories: lean meat, medium-fat meat, and high-fat meat. One ounce (one meat exchange) of each of these includes:

	CARBOHYDRATE (grams)	PROTEIN (grams)	FAT (grams)	CALORIES
Lean	0	7	3	55
Medium-fat	0	7	5	75
High-fat	0	7	8	100

You are encouraged to use more lean and medium-fat meat, poultry, and fish in your meal plan. This will help decrease your fat intake, which may help decrease your risk for heart disease. The items from the high-fat group are high in saturated fat, cholesterol, and calories. You should limit your choices from the high-fat group to three (3) times per week. Meat and substitutes do not contribute any fiber to your meal plan. Meats and meat substitutes that have 400 milligrams or more of sodium per exchange are footnoted. Meats and meat substitutes that have 400 milligrams or more of sodium if two or more exchanges are eaten are footnoted.

TIPS

1. Bake, roast, broil, grill, or boil these foods rather than frying them with added fat.
2. Use a nonstick pan spray or a nonstick pan to brown or fry these foods.
3. Trim off visible fat before and after cooking.
4. Do not add flour, bread crumbs, coating mixes, or fat to these foods when preparing them.
5. Weight meat after removing bones and fat, and after cooking. Three ounces of cooked meat is about equal to 4 ounces of raw meat. Some examples of meat portions are:

> 2 ounces meat (2 meat exchanges) =
> 1 small chicken leg or thigh
> ½ cup cottage cheese or tuna
> 3 ounces meat (3 meat exchanges) =
> 1 medium pork chop

        1 small hamburger
        ½ of a whole chicken breast
        1 unbreaded fish fillet
        cooked meat, about the size of a deck of cards

6. Restaurants usually serve prime cuts of meat, which are high in fat and calories.

LEAN MEAT AND SUBSTITUTES

(One exchange is equal to any one of the following items.)

BEEF:	USDA Good or Choice grades of lean beef, such as round, sirloin, and flank steak; tenderloin; and chipped beef*	1 oz.
PORK:	Lean pork, such as fresh ham; canned, cured, or boiled ham*, Canadian bacon*, tenderloin	1 oz.
VEAL:	All cuts are lean except for veal cutlets (ground or cubed). Examples of lean veal are chops and roasts.	1 oz.
POULTRY:	Chicken, turkey, Cornish hen (without skin)	1 oz.
FISH:	All fresh and frozen fish	1 oz.
	Crab, lobster, scallops, shrimp, clams (fresh or canned in water)	2 oz.
	Oysters	6 medium
	Tuna** (canned in water)	¼ cup
	Herring** (uncreamed or smoked)	1 oz.
	Sardines (canned)	2 medium
WILDGAME:	Venison, rabbit, squirrel	1 oz.
	Pheasant, duck, goose (without skin)	1 oz.
CHEESE:	Any cottage cheese**	¼ cup
	Grated Parmesan	2 Tbsp.
	Diet cheeses* (with less than 55 calories per ounce)	1 oz.

OTHER: 95% fat-free luncheon meat*   1½ oz.
Egg whites   3 whites
Egg substitues (with less than 55   ½ cup
calories per ½ cup)

*400 milligrams or more of sodium per exchange.
**400 milligrams or more of sodium if two or more exchanges are
eaten.

MEDIUM-FAT MEAT AND SUBSTITUTES

(One exchange is equal to any one of the following items.)

BEEF: Most beef products fall into this category.   1 oz.
Examples are all ground beef, roast (rib,
chuck, rump), steak (cubed, Porterhouse,
T-bone), and meat loaf.

PORK: Most pork products fall into this category.   1 oz.
Examples are chops, loin roast, Boston butt,
and cutlets.

LAMB: Most lamb products fall into this category.   1 oz.
Examples are chops, leg, and roast.

VEAL: Cutlet (ground or cubed, unbreaded)   1 oz.

POULTRY: Chicken (with skin), domestic duck or goose   1 oz.
(well drained of fat), ground turkey

FISH: Tuna* (canned in oil and drained)   ¼ cup
Salmon* (canned)   ¼ cup

CHEESE: Skim or part-skim milk cheeses, such as: ¼ cup
Ricotta
Mozzarella   1 oz.
Diet cheeses** (with 56–80 calories per   1 oz.
ounce)

*400 milligrams or more of sodium if two or more exchanges are
eaten.
**400 milligrams or more of sodium per exchange.

OTHER:	86% fat-free luncheon meat*	1 oz.
	Egg high in cholesterol, limit to 3 per week	1
	Egg substitutes (with 56–80 calories per ¼ cup)	¼ cup
	Tofu (2½ in. × 2¾ in. × 1 in.)	4 oz.
	Liver, heart, kidney, sweetbreads (high in cholesterol)	1 oz.

*400 milligrams or more of sodium if two or more exchanges are eaten.

**400 miligrams or more of sodium per exchange.

HIGH-FAT MEAT AND SUBSTITUTES

Remember, these items are high in saturated fat, cholesterol, and calories and should be used only three (3) times per week.

(One exchange is equal to any one of the following items.)

BEEF:	Most USDA Prime cuts of beef, such as ribs, corned beef*	1 oz.
PORK:	Spareribs, ground pork, port sausage** (patty or link)	1 oz.
LAMB:	Patties (ground lamb)	1 oz.
FISH:	Any fried fish product	1 oz.
CHEESE:	All regular cheeses, such as American**, blue**, Cheddar*, Monterey Jack*, Swiss	1 oz.
OTHER:	Luncheon meat**, such as bologna, salami, pimiento loaf	1 oz.
	Sausage**, such as Polish, Italian smoked	1 oz.
	Knockwurst**	1 oz.
	Bratwurst*	1 oz.
	Frankfurter** (turkey or chicken)	1 frank (10/lb.)
	Peanut butter (contains unsaturated fat)	1 Tbsp.

Count as one high-fat meat plus one fat exchange:

Frankfurter** (beef, pork, or com-   1 frank (10/lb.)
bination)

*400 milligrams or more of sodium if two or more exchanges are eaten.

**400 milligrams or more of sodium per exchange.

3 VEGETABLE LIST

Each vegetable serving on this list contains about 5 grams of carbohydrate, 2 grams of protein, and 25 calories. Vegetables contain 2 to 3 grams of dietary fiber. Vegetables that contain 400 milligrams or more of sodium per exchange are footnoted.

Vegetables are a good source of vitamins and minerals. Fresh and frozen vegetables have more vitamins and less added salt. Rinsing canned vegetables will remove much of the salt.

Unless otherwise noted, the serving size for vegetables (one vegetable exchange) is:

+ ½ cup of cooked vegetables or vegetable juice
+ 1 cup of raw vegetables

Artichoke (½ medium)   Greens (collard, mustard,
Asparagus   turnip)
Bean sprouts   Kohlrabi
Beans (green, wax, Italian)   Leeks
Beets   Mushrooms, cooked
Broccoli   Okra
Brussels sprouts   Onions
Cabbage, cooked   Pea pods
Carrots   Peppers (green)
Cauliflower   Rutabaga
Eggplant   Sauerkraut*

(continued on page 370)

Spinach, cooked
Summer squash (crookneck)
Tomato (one large)
Tomato/vegetable juice*

Turnips
Water chestnuts
Zucchini, cooked

Starchy vegetables such as corn, peas, and potatoes are found on the Starch/Bread List. For free vegetables, see Free Food List on page 376.

*400 milligrams or more of sodium per exchange.

4 FRUIT LIST

Each item on this list contains about 15 grams of carbohydrate and 60 calories. Fresh, frozen, and dried fruits have about 2 grams of fiber per exchange. Fruits that have 3 or more grams of fiber per exchange are footnoted. Fruit juices contain very little dietary fiber.

The carbohydrate and calorie contents for a fruit exchange are based on the usual serving of the most commonly eaten fruits. Use fresh fruits or fruits frozen or canned without sugar added. Whole fruit is more filling than fruit juice and may be a better choice for those who are trying to lose weight. Unless otherwise noted, the serving size for one fruit exchange is:

+ ½ cup of fresh fruit or fruit juice
+ ¼ cup of dried fruit

FRESH, FROZEN AND UNSWEETENED CANNED FRUIT

Apple (raw, 2 in. across)	1 apple
Applesauce (unsweetened)	½ cup
Apricots (medium or raw)	4 apricots
Apricots (canned)	½ cup or 4 halves
Banana (9 in. long)	½ banana
Blackberries* (raw)	¾ cup

Blueberries* (raw)	¾ cup
Cantaloupe (5 in. across)	⅓ melon
(cubes)	1 cup
Cherries (large, raw)	12 cherries
Cherries (canned)	½ cup
Figs (raw, 2 in. across)	2 figs
Fruit cocktail (canned)	½ cup
Grapefruit (medium)	½ grapefruit
Grapefruit (segments)	¾ cup
Grapes (small)	15 grapes
Honeydew melon	
(medium)	⅛ melon
(cubes)	1 cup
Kiwi (large)	1 kiwi
Mandarin oranges	¾ cup
Mango (small)	½ mango
Nectarine* (2½ in. across)	1 nectarine
Orange (2½ in. across)	1 orange
Papaya	1 cup
Peach (2¾ in. across)	1 peach, or ¾ cup
Peaches (canned)	½ cup, or 2 halves
Pear	½ large, or 1 small
Pears (canned)	½ cup, or 2 halves
Persimmon (medium, native)	2 persimmons
Pineapple (raw)	¾ cup
Pineapple (canned)	⅓ cup
Plum (raw, 2 in. across)	2 plums
Pomegranate*	½ pomegranate
Raspberries* (raw)	1 cup
Strawberries* (raw, whole)	1¼ cups
Tangerine* (2½ in. across)	2 tangerines
Watermelon (cubes)	1¼ cups

*3 grams or more of fiber per exchange.

DRIED FRUIT

Apples*	4 rings
Apricots*	7 halves
Dates	2½ medium
Figs*	1½
Prunes*	3 medium
Raisins	2 Tbsp.

*3 grams or more of fiber per exchange.

FRUIT JUICE

Apple juice/cider	½ cup
Cranberry juice cocktail	⅓ cup
Grape juice	⅓ cup
Grapefruit juice	½ cup
Orange juice	½ cup
Pineapple juice	½ cup
Prune juice	⅓ cup

5 MILK LIST

Each serving of milk or milk products on this list contains about 12 grams of carbohydrate and 8 grams of protein. The amount of fat in milk is measured in percent (%) of butterfat. The calories vary, depending on what kind of milk you choose. The list is divided into three parts based on the amount of fat and calories: skim/very low-fat milk, low-fat milk, and whole milk. One serving (one milk exchange) of each of these includes:

	CARBOHYDRATE (*grams*)	PROTEIN (*grams*)	FAT (*grams*)	CALORIES
Skim/Very Low-fat	12	8	trace	90
Low-fat	12	8	5	120
Whole	12	8	8	150

Milk is the body's main source of calcium, the mineral needed for growth and repair of bones. Yogurt is also a good source of calcium. Yogurt and many dry or powdered milk products have different amounts of fat. If you have questions about a particular item, read the label to find out the fat and calorie content.

Milk is good to drink, but it can also be added to cereal, and to other foods. Many tasty dishes, such as sugar-free pudding, are made with milk (see the Combination Foods List on pages 377–379). Add life to plain yogurt by adding one of your fruit exchanges to it.

SKIM AND VERY LOW-FAT MILK

Skim milk	1 cup
½% milk	1 cup
1% milk	1 cup
Low-fat buttermilk	1 cup
Evaporated skim milk	½ cup
Dry nonfat milk	⅓ cup
Plain nonfat yogurt	8 oz.

LOW-FAT MILK

2% milk	1 cup
Plain low-fat yogurt (with added nonfat milk solids)	8 oz.

WHOLE MILK

The whole milk group has much more fat per serving than the skim and low-fat groups. Whole milk has more than 3¼% butterfat. Try to limit your choices from the whole milk group as much as possible.

Whole milk	1 cup
Evaporated whole milk	½ cup
Whole plain yogurt	8 oz.

6 FAT LIST

Each serving on the fat list contains about 5 grams of fat and 45 calories.

The foods on the fat list contain mostly fat, although some items may also contain a small amount of protein. All fats are high in calories and should be carefully measured. Everyone should modify fat intake by eating unsaturated fats instead of saturated fats. The sodium content of these foods varies widely. Check the label for sodium information.

UNSATURATED FATS

Avocado	⅛ medium
Margarine	1 tsp.
Margarine*, diet	1 Tbsp.
Mayonnaise	1 tsp.
Mayonnaise*, reduced-calorie	1 Tbsp.
Nuts and Seeds:	
Almonds, dry roasted	6 whole
Cashews, dry roasted	1 Tbsp.
Pecans	2 whole
Peanuts	20 small or 10 large
Walnuts	2 whole
Other nuts	1 Tbsp.
Seeds, pine nuts, sunflower (without shells)	1 Tbsp.
Pumpkin seeds	2 tsp.
Oil (corn, cottonseed, safflower, soybean, sunflower, olive, peanut)	1 tsp.
Olives*	10 small or 5 large
Salad dressing, mayonnaise-type	2 tsp.
Salad dressing, mayonnaise-type, reduced-calorie	1 Tbsp.

| Salad dressing* (oil varieties) | 1 Tbsp. |
| Salad dressing**, reduced-calorie | 2 Tbsp. |

SATURATED FATS

Bacon*	1 slice
Butter	1 tsp.
Chitterlings	½ ounce
Coconut, shredded	2 Tbsp.
Coffee whitener, liquid	2 Tbsp.
Coffee whitener, powder	4 tsp.
Cream (light, coffee, table)	2 Tbsp.
Cream (heavy, whipping)	1 Tbsp.
Cream, sour	2 Tbsp.
Cream cheese	1 Tbsp.
Salt pork*	¼ ounce

*400 milligrams or more of sodium if two or more exchanges are eaten.

**400 milligrams or more of sodium per exchange.

FREE FOODS

A free food is any food or drink that contains less than 20 calories per serving. You can eat as much as you want of those items that have no serving size specified. You may eat two or three servings per day of those items that have a specific servings size. Be sure to spread them out through the day.

DRINKS:

Bouillon* or broth without fat
Bouillon, low-sodium
Carbonated drink, sugar-free
Carbonated water
Club soda

Cocoa powder, unsweetened (1 Tbsp.)
Coffee / Tea
Drink mixes, sugar-free
Tonic water, sugar-free

NONSTICK PAN SPRAY

FRUIT

Cranberries, unsweetened (½ cup)
Rhubarb, unsweetened (½ cup)

VEGETABLES

(raw, 1 cup)

Cabbage
Celery
Chinese cabbage*
Cucumber
Green onion
Hot peppers
Mushrooms
Radishes
Zucchini*

SALAD GREENS

Endive
Escarole
Lettuce
Romaine
Spinach

SWEET SUBSTITUTES

Candy, hard, sugar-free
Gelatin, sugar-free
Gum, sugar-free
Jam/Jelly, sugar-free (less than 20 cal./2 tsp.)
Pancake syrup, sugar-free (1–2 Tbsp.)
Sugar substitues (saccharin, aspartame)
Whipped topping (2 Tbsp.)

CONDIMENTS

     Catsup (1 Tbsp.)
     Horseradish
     Mustard
     Pickles**, dill, unsweetened
     Salad dressing, low-calorie (2 Tbsp.)
     Taco sauce (3 Tbsp.)
     Vinegar

*3 grams or more of fiber per exchange.
**400 milligrams or more of sodium per exchange.

Seasonings can be very helpful in making food taste better. Be careful of how much sodium you use. Read the label, choose those seasonings that do not contain sodium or salt.

Basil (fresh)	Garlic	Paprika
Celery seeds	Garlic powder	Pepper
Chili powder	Herbs	Pimento
Chives	Hot pepper sauce	Soy sauce*
Cinnamon	Lemon	Soy sauce*, low-sodium ("lite")
Curry	Lemon juice	
Dill	Lemon pepper	Spices
Flavoring extracts (vanilla, almond, walnut, peppermint, butter, lemon, etc.)	Lime	Wine, used in cooking (¼ cup)
	Lime juice	Worcestershire sauce
	Mint	
	Onion powder	
	Oregano	

*400 milligrams or more of sodium per exchange.

COMBINATION FOODS

Much of the food we eat is mixed together in various combinations. These combination foods do not fit into only one exchange list. It can be quite hard to tell what is in a certain casserole or baked food item. This is a list of average values for some typical combination foods. This list will help you fit these foods into your meal plan. Ask your dietitian for information about any other foods you'd like to eat. The *American Diabetes Association/ American Dietetic Family Cookbooks* and the *American Diabetes Association Holiday Cookbook* have many recipes and further information about many foods, including combination foods. Check your library or local bookstore.

FOOD	AMOUNT	EXCHANGES
Casseroles, homemade	1 cup (8 oz.)	2 starch, 2 medium-fat meat, 1 fat
Cheese pizza*, thin crust	¼ of 15 oz. or ¼ of 10"	2 starch, 1 medium-fat meat, 1 fat
Chili with bean* ** (commercial)	1 cup (8 oz.)	2 starch, 2 medium-fat meat, 2 fat
Chow mein* (without noodles or rice)	2 cups (16 oz.)	1 starch, 2 vegetable, 2 lean meat
Macaroni and cheese*	1 cup (8 oz.)	2 starch, 1 medium-fat meat, 2 fat
Soup		
Bean* **	1 cup (8 oz.)	1 starch, 1 vegetable, 1 lean meat
Chunky, all varieties*	10 ¾ oz. can	1 starch, 1 vegetable, 1 medium-fat meat

Cream* (made with water)	1 cup (8 oz.)	1 starch, 1 fat
Vegetable* or broth-type*	1 cup (8 oz.)	1 starch
Spaghetti and meatballs* (canned)	1 cup (8 oz.)	2 starch, 1 medium-fat meat, 1 fat
Sugar-free pudding (made with skim milk)	½ cup	1 starch

If beans are used as a meat substitute

Dried beans**, peas**, lentils**	1 cup (cooked)	2 starch, 1 lean meat

*400 milligrams or more of sodium per exchange.
**3 grams or more of fiber per exchange.

FOODS FOR OCCASIONAL USE

Moderate amounts of some foods can be used in your meal plan, in spite of their sugar or fat content, as long as you can maintain blood-glucose control. The following list includes average exchange values for some of those foods. Because they are concentrated sources of carbohydrate, you will notice that the portion sizes are very small. Check with your dietitian for advice on how often and when you can eat them.

FOOD	AMOUNT	EXCHANGES
Angel food cake	¹⁄₁₂ cake	2 starch
Cake, no icing	¹⁄₁₂ cake, or a 3″ square	2 starch, 2 fat
Cookies	2 small (1¾″ across)	1 starch, 1 fat
Frozen fruit yogurt	⅓ cup	1 starch
Gingersnaps	3	1 starch

(continued on page 380)

Granola	¼ cup	1 starch, 1 fat
Granola bars	1 small	1 starch, 1 fat
Ice cream, any flavor	½ cup	1 starch, 2 fat
Ice milk, any flavor	½ cup	1 starch, 1 fat
Sherbet, any flavor	¼ cup	1 starch
Snack chips*, all varieties	1 oz.	1 starch, 2 fat
Vanilla wafers	6 small	1 starch

*400 milligrams or more of sodium if two or more exchanges are eaten.

Index